Copyright © 2023 by Transformation Global Inc.

All rights reserved. No part of this book may be reproduced, stored in a retrieval system, or transmitted in any form or by any means, electronic, mechanical, photocopying, recording, or otherwise, without the prior written permission of the publisher, except in the case of brief quotations embodied in critical reviews and certain other noncommercial uses permitted by copyright law.

Disclaimer:
While Dr. Maggie Yu is a medical doctor, the content in this book should not be construed as medical advice or as a substitute for professional medical diagnosis, consultation, or treatment. For questions regarding your medical condition(s), please consult your physician or another qualified health provider. Never disregard professional medical advice or delay in seeking because of something you have read in this book.

Published by Transformation Global Inc.
23505 E. Appleway Ave. Suite 200
Liberty Lake, WA 99019
United States
www.8OutoftheBox.com

Printed in USA

ISBN: 979-8-9890317-8-8

# BOOK BONUS BUNDLE
## (VALUED AT OVER $597)

3 Bonus Items:

- Hormone Certainty Course (5-Part Video Training + Workbook)

  ▶ Uncover the surprising truth about hormone-related symptoms with Dr. Maggie's guidance in Transform's Hormone Certainty Online Training Course. Explore hormonally vulnerable times in your life, map your hormone timeline, and tackle complex multi-system symptoms like pain, fatigue, insomnia, IBS, and anxiety. Be amazed by effective, immediate steps to alleviate your symptoms and discover actionable strategies to balance your hormones from Dr. Maggie's expert insights.

- Insider's Guide: How to Transform Your Thyroid

  ▶ Dive into the transformative world of thyroid health with Dr. Maggie's guide, How to Transform Your Thyroid. Unlock the secrets to protecting and optimizing your thyroid for better overall well-being, uncover enlightening thyroid training, find solutions to pressing questions, and access a comprehensive symptom checklist. Take immediate action to shield and optimize your thyroid through expert-proven steps.

- Mast Cell Activation Syndrome Training Course (3-part video course)

  ▶ Unlock solutions for food reactions and allergies with our exclusive Histamine Intolerance and MCAS training. Gain control of your health through our FREE 3-step training series, learning to support your immune system, identify triggering foods, and manage symptoms effectively. Experience dietary freedom and expert strategies to conquer allergies and gut inflammation, ensuring a worry-free life for you and your family.

## PRAISE FOR DR. MAGGIE

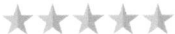

"Dr. Maggie Yu is an expert in autoimmune, hormones, gut health, and chronic diseases. She's not just looking to treat the symptoms, which is what most doctors do, but she gets to the root cause of disease to address the source issue."

- Kevin Harrington
the Original Shark from Shark Tank

"Simple tools, steps, and strategies are laid out in this book that will change the way you care for and know yourself. In a symptom-focused medical world, finding a like-minded educator like Dr. Maggie Yu who directly addresses the root cause of so many disorders and diseases is like finding a needle in a haystack."

- Sue Hitzmann, creator of MELT Method

"Dr. Maggie is fierce in her passion...educating her patients. Her humor is infectious. The amazing gift I got was the understanding of what might be causing my symptoms and what I needed to do to fix it. Knowledge is power, and that is what Dr. Maggie drills down in all of us. Thank you for sharing all the pearls you gathered through your own difficult times."

- Arti Bhan-Kachroo, Dentist

*"As a journalist, I'm a thorough researcher, and that's how I found Dr. Maggie. I was looking for medical answers for myself, answers no other doctor could seem to provide. Dr. Maggie has a vast collection of trainings on YouTube, in podcasts, and in her Facebook community, and what I learned from her was groundbreaking. I decided to work directly with her in one of her programs. Dr. Maggie, her programs, and now her book present a paradigm-challenging system for both conventional care and functional medicine care for hard-to-treat chronic diseases. I myself have watched and also interviewed many who have utilized the Transform system to turn around countless symptoms and diagnoses that conventional medicine had deemed to be untreatable. This book encapsulates 8 great lessons I wish everyone knew about, including me, early in their health journey."*

- Anne Imanuel, TV News Anchor and Host

*"I was sick for almost 20 years with terrible migraines, allergies, random hives, dizziness, terrible fatigue, weird reactions, and feelings every time I ate, horrible periods; the list goes on and on. I am an RN, and I learned a TON. They do not teach professionals this stuff."*

- Amie Staberg-Biebl, Registered Nurse

I dedicate this book to Jonathan,
My best friend and partner, the one who was there to restore my
faith in humanity.

For
Tao Han
Emma
The two who always provided me with focus

In celebration of
The tens of thousands of patients and clients I've been blessed to work with, and whose stories and transformations have inspired my work and this book. You have been my greatest teachers.

Thankful for
The hard-working men and women on the Transform & MY.MD team, and Deb Law, for your encouragement and support with this book.

# TABLE OF CONTENTS

01  Introduction

15  How to Use this Book

20  Lesson 1: Leading with Curiosity

43  Lesson 2: Digestion - The First Domino

77  Lesson 3: The Gut: Getting Off the Merry-Go-Round

109  Lesson 4: Certainty About Food is Required

131  Lesson 5: Blood Sugar Mastery

173  Lesson 6: It's Just Your Hormones... It Can't Be Your Hormones

207  Lesson 7: Creating Experiences for Your Health Transformation

223  Lesson 8: Mindset to Mind Growth

246  Conclusion

251  About Maggie Yu MD IFMCP

253  Experiences Available Through Transform

260  Appendix

264  Recipes

273  Glossary

280  Personal Action Plan

**8 Out of the Box Ways to Transform Your Health**
From Confusion to Confidence: The Playbook for Whole Body Wellness

# INTRODUCTION

In a world where I was trained to have answers, my own health became the question mark I couldn't escape. My days were filled with patient charts and diagnoses, yet the most perplexing case was the one I couldn't chart: my own.

When I graduated from medical school, I was certain I had become a healer and doctor. I became a family physician for the next ten years and knew I was doing a good job. On the outside, I was successful professionally. I graduated in the top 2% of my class in medical school at UCLA. I loved my family medicine residency. I was married with my first child on the way when I started my first job with Kaiser Permanente nearly 25 years ago. Yet, there were frays.

By all accounts, I was a well-loved and high-performing family practitioner. I loved my job as a medical director of a large clinic, teaching and managing other doctors and staff. I loved being a doctor. However, my own health puzzle and frustrations were spilling into my work and care of patients. I could no longer separate my physical and mental health struggles from my professional self.

The birth of my first child led to a series of health mysteries no one could solve. I had severe postpartum depression, mastitis (infection in the breast), and an antibiotic-induced infection called C. difficile. I was feeling worse every day throughout my body. Yet, all of my bloodwork was normal. None of the rounds of treatment helped me. These health symptoms culminated into yet new symptoms when my second child was born. I developed insulin-dependent diabetes during my second pregnancy and ongoing chronic fatigue, weight gain, and hair loss issues. At the age of 36, I went into full-blown early menopause, and yet, no one knew why.

I had severe fibromyalgia (which most doctors then and now don't believe is real) and chronic pain in my elbows, jaw, and back. I had neuropathy and nerve-related pain in my low back going down my left hip and leg. I was gaining weight and losing hair, and I couldn't sleep. For nearly a decade, I slept less than 3 hours a night. I attributed it to stress from a huge patient load, clinical management responsibilities, and a failing marriage.

I felt alone. I was disconnected from my body, soul, and the world around me. The loneliest times were in the middle of the night when I couldn't sleep. When my then-husband came to bed, I would pretend to be asleep. Yet, I would lay awake all night, feeling alone, scared, and shut down. I thought, "Isn't this how everyone feels in their thirties?"

To add insult to injury, mysterious symptoms kept emerging: why was I losing my edge, focus, and mind? Why do I feel like I have Attention Deficit Disorder (ADD)?

How did I get diagnosed with it in my late 30s?

Now, not only am I on antidepressants but also ADD medications and a slew of other medications I prescribe my patients all the time. I prided myself on remembering fine details about my patients, yet I struggled with numbers and dates.

I was feeling sick, physically and emotionally. I knew I wasn't well. But I thought I was expected to be feeling great. Another driving force was that I didn't want to be a failure. I had never been someone who failed in whatever my goals were. I did not want to be a failure to my parents, family, or my patients. The disparity between what was on the outside and what was happening inside created feelings of guilt and shame. I judged myself by thinking, "You shouldn't feel this way." Deny, reject, delay.

I got physically so sick that it impacted me professionally. I lost myself, my job, and my marriage. I hit rock bottom. There is something about the bottom and those moments of darkness that laid the foundation for how I started to get better. I could have died. I got close. I could have given up. I didn't. Something in me knew that this wasn't it. There must be something I'm missing that I'm not seeing. What was I not seeing?

One early morning, sitting on the bathroom floor crying quietly to myself, I had a revelation. There's something about rock bottom that helps you realize doing something, anything different, would be a step up and out. If I wanted something this big to change, I had to do it by thinking and doing something differently to get a new outcome. I didn't know how. I didn't have anyone to

**8 Out of the Box Ways to Transform Your Health**
From Confusion to Confidence: The Playbook for Whole Body Wellness

ask. Oh, how I wish 25 years ago, there was a Dr. Maggie to ask, hey, what did you do? So, I had to conjure her. I had to manifest her. I had to take the first steps to find my own solutions. I visualized and saw who Maggie was: healed, happy, excited, and in love with life. I thought, what are some of the first steps it would take or even just the next step, thought, or action I would have to take to step towards her?

And I did. It was hard at first. It took work. But when you start to love something, it no longer is work. It becomes a passion. It started with that first decision and finding that first domino. I attended a training on the thyroid from a chiropractor who had written an incredible book. The science he was teaching and the scientific sense it made was exciting. I learned about the hundreds of studies behind everything he was saying. There was data and evidence for a totally different approach to the thyroid. And I discovered I did actually have a thyroid problem, an autoimmune disease of the thyroid called Hashimoto's that no one, including myself, knew was a major root cause of my early menopause and other symptoms.

I decided to open my own practice. Because of my early menopause, I had embarked on learning everything I could on how to test, balance, and prescribe hormones. The clinic exploded, focusing at first on testing and balancing hormones. I had to hire additional providers. In Portland, partnering with a naturopathic school, I found a great one to work with me in my clinic to become our naturopathic medical director. She's an incredible hormone expert and added so much to my education.

8 Out of the Box Ways to Transform Your Health
From Confusion to Confidence: The Playbook for Whole Body Wellness

The clinic offered primary care and natural medicine care. We grew to eight providers, with half of them being naturopathic doctors and the other half conventionally trained providers.

A learning environment for medical providers to learn holistic or natural medicine, without a significant investment of both time and money to attend another six years of education, which didn't exist at the time. And naturopathic physicians had little opportunity to be trained in a real-life medical clinic or hospital setting. I created a learning environment where we learned from each other. We presented cases to explore how we can combine conventional and holistic medicine in our approach to patient care. We worked side-by-side with most of our patients. We learned, and the clinic grew. In those eight years, I embarked on hundreds of hours every year to attend conferences to meet and find hundreds of colleagues in all branches of holistic medicine to learn from and collaborate with.

As I learned, my world grew, the number of people around me grew, and I got better. I took every part of me that was broken, and I figured out how to get the best of both worlds to heal myself. Piece by piece, I mended myself.

The Japanese have a word, Kintsugi. It means golden repair. Kintsugi is the process by which broken ceramics are repaired with lacquered gold. The result is a sealed piece with gold seams where the cracks were. The final product is a repaired piece that is waterproof and strong yet infinitely more beautiful in its repaired brokenness.

That's what happened to me. My health journey and aloneness broke me. It broke me a thousand ways with a thousand cuts. But piece by piece, through thinking differently and doing differently, these individual strands of knowledge and wisdom repaired each crack with gold. I healed myself. And over the next decade, I took that hard-earned wisdom and never looked back. I began to teach not only the naturopathic and medical providers in my clinic, but we began to take an educational approach to our patients who were used to conventional medicine. We had to teach them how diet, hormones, lifestyle, food, and movement mattered. We provided educational opportunities to patients and our colleagues. While other clinics focused on the churn, we focused on educating people. That took time, but seeing the lightbulb and the ability of people to access the vast range of tools we were able to offer fueled my desire forever to be a teacher first and a doctor second.

As a teacher, I taught my patients how to think differently, do differently, and, as a result, get out-of-the-box results. I spent the years that followed building an online community and online educational programs with live teaching and advice to patients and providers. I started a supplement company focused on educating people on the why behind supplementation. I speak and write about functional medicine (a combination of convention and holistic medicine) through my podcasts, YouTube channels, and other social media outlets. I have been interviewed to teach on autoimmunity, hormone balance, and mindset growth work and have taught at conferences.

This book is the culmination and a roadmap of some of the most important things I had to think differently about. In order to create this roadmap and the turning point of my story, I had to realize that the system I had learned to operate in was inherently flawed and broken. In my own learning and healing journey, I've evolved into a teaching journey. The teacher has arrived. Is the student ready?

## Why You Should Read This Book

**When a student is ready, the teacher appears.** I was experiencing my own health and professional crisis during much of my early career. I had to become an avid student, and when I was ready, my teachers appeared. I share some of the teachers and what I've learned with you in the lessons in this book.

Instead of being the good family medicine doctor who just told people what to do, which was faster and easier, I challenged myself to teach in my one-on-one interactions. The biggest challenge was learning to teach by writing and on video through social media. I started with a 30-day challenge to teach something every day for thirty days on Facebook. Those weren't pretty, but they are still up on social media. When I look back at those, I see an eager and excited Dr. Maggie learning the skill of teaching on live video. I'm proud of her. She wasn't afraid to do something different. At the end of thirty days, I didn't stop. I kept going. The regular live teaching on Facebook and YouTube grew and is still going strong six years later. The online community Facebook group is 92,229 and growing! The students found me.

Teaching in person and online has become a passion and superpower. Lao Tzu says, "When a student is ready, the teacher appears." I am still a doctor, but I consider my true vocation to be that of a teacher. My invitation to you is: there's a reason you're reading this book; you are ready.

This book is me sharing some of the best of what I've taught with the world. It is concise, action steps oriented, and focused. When you read this book, you will understand why anything and everything is happening in your body. These lessons will connect many of these dots for you. The ability to connect the dots with disparate symptoms and diagnoses is the modern health plague. The best solution for that is for those who have made those connections to show others how to do that.

**Great lessons save you time.** The usual timeline of someone getting sick with one symptom, waiting a few weeks or months for a doctor's visit, getting testing, reviewing results, getting a prescription, and then it doesn't work. Wait six weeks to go back to the doctor, get another test, try another drug, and get another referral. That's just one symptom. For example, even if you saw one of your doctors for fifteen minutes every six weeks for a year, you would not be able to match just one week of the amount of time our clients work with me and my team. In the average week, our clients directly learn and work with us for about six hours a week. That amount of focus and learning cannot happen in a clinical setting, even over a two-year time frame.

How about if it's easier than that? What if you could learn one answer by reading one chapter in this book? Let me be your teacher through these pages.

It's my intention when I teach that I save people a tremendous amount of time to get from sick to great. What you will find is that by reading the book, you decrease and compress the amount of time it takes you to get better. Anytime you have a result you want, it takes time, money, and effort. Time is the only resource in there that you cannot get back. So, finding teachers, doctors, and mentors who provide great lessons saves you the time it takes to get a result. It also drastically reduces the time you have to suffer. Find great teachers, learn great lessons, and compress the amount of time it takes for you to get better. That's why you should read this book.

Why else should you read this book?

**Realize that you're not alone.** I felt I was alone on my health journey. Like a frog unaware of the gradually heating water, our health issues often escalate without immediate recognition. Things build: a headache here, or you struggle to remember a detail you should have no problem recalling. The whole time, the temperature is rising, and the struggle is getting more and more intense. Many one-on-one visits to various doctors and specialists punctuate this journey. And the rest of the time, most of us are on the internet trying to figure out what's going on. These are very solitary activities.

8 Out of the Box Ways to Transform Your Health
From Confusion to Confidence: The Playbook for Whole Body Wellness

When we feel misunderstood, not heard, and not seen in the healthcare system, many of us detach or withdraw. Many people give up. As symptoms mount and solutions fade, it becomes a very isolating, lonely journey. One of the most important reasons to read this book is to realize that you are not alone. There are tens of thousands of people just like you with the symptoms you have and the lack of answers you've had to deal with. Every time I talk to someone who's seen one of the case studies on our YouTube channel or has heard my story, the most common response is, "Thank goodness for that story; it made me realize that I wasn't alone."

Discovering that you're not alone carries immense transformative power. It's a revelation that can provide solace, validation, and a renewed sense of hope. When you realize that others have faced similar challenges or experienced the same emotions, it can be incredibly comforting. This shared connection reminds us that our struggles, joys, and triumphs are part of a collective human experience.

My story and the case studies shared within this book are a testament to our shared human experiences. If you're seeking more, we have hundreds of case studies on our YouTube channel. Moreover, our dedicated team has invested significant efforts to cultivate and support an empowering Facebook community. At the time of writing this book, we have 92,229 members, reflecting a widespread consensus on the importance of unity and mutual support. If you've ever felt isolated in your journey, let these stories reassure you: you are not alone. We're here, standing beside you.

**Know that you're not a unicorn. Your problems can be fixed.** I share many stories in this book to highlight some of the very typical symptoms, diagnoses, and health patterns that show up all the time. It's in shining the light on these stories that I want you to realize you're not alone. However, even when people know they're not alone, when they haven't been listened to, they begin to feel like they have a unique problem that no one can help with.

It's what I call "I'm a super special rare zebra that can't be helped" syndrome. There were many points in my health journey where I thought I had a rare, undiagnosable condition that no one else had ever seen and that I would never be able to get better. That's bleak, and that's hopeless. But visit after visit, test after test, drug after drug, and night after night of feeling miserable becomes living proof that I can't be helped.

The belief that I have a rare, incurable condition that no one can help becomes a powerful story and identity. Ben, a client I worked with, shared openly that he has lived with being a sick person with an incurable form of anxiety that reacts to every medication or supplement violently. As a result of this belief, he refuses all medications or supplements. He realized that just the idea of putting a supplement or new food near his mouth elicited severe nausea and rapid heart rate. His belief that his problem could never be fixed, along with his belief that he has a rare, incurable disease, caused him to be his own obstacle to wellness. His sick story has become a familiar story. He found comfort in its familiarity. However, this story no longer served him and is now keeping him closed to new ideas and becoming the thing that was keeping him sick.

His fear.

Ben shared that one of the things that gave him the most courage was seeing other people who had very similar problems. He learned that many people thought they had extremely rare forms of diseases. He learned that they and he had a root cause that was in these lessons. He witnessed them making changes and taking a dietary change or taking a supplement they needed, and they got better. He got confirmation that their problem could be fixed, which helped him build confidence in his new belief that his problem could absolutely be fixed. He became courageous as a result of community, and he took that courage to build new beliefs and stories that serve him. He is not an unusually rare zebra; he experienced fear, doubt, and paralysis as many people do. However, he realized that he now had a choice. He saw evidence to bolster the belief that he's not incurable and, in fact, he holds the keys to his own freedom. If Ben reminds you of something in yourself, you now have a choice. Are you ready to believe that you could be helped? It's only when you can see, feel, and taste that future that transformation can exist.

This book is peppered with real-life case studies, and you will see yourself in many of them. You will know you're not alone, and what you're experiencing isn't all that rare. People like you and sicker than you get better every day. I know because I work with them and interview them every week. This fact will motivate and mobilize you into a state of excitement, hope, and curiosity to want to learn: how did they do that? The answers are in the lessons.

**Learn how to think outside the box to get different results!** In the eight lessons, I've shared some of the top ways to think about problems differently. If how you and your doctor have thought about this problem has already led to solutions and permanent results, you wouldn't need to look at other solutions. That's why you should read this and get other solutions. So read it expecting to challenge and question you and your doctor's thoughts and assumptions about your health problem. Have an excited and open learner's mind. Often, the solution to the problem is something you haven't seen or thought of before. The lesson about Leading with Curiosity should be the first lesson to read. My curiosity led me to learn everything I know now. So, with an open mind and an open heart, let's get out of the box and into a world of infinite answers and solutions.

Whether you feel overwhelmed, frustrated, or hopeless, know that there is help for you in the following pages. That is my promise.

## Action Steps

1. Join our 92,229 and growing Facebook community, "Transform Your Health Naturally," to directly engage with the community, my team, and me. www.DrMaggieYu.com/Transform
2. Check out our entire library on our YouTube channel for a full playlist of case studies and trainings. www.youtube.com/@DrMaggieYu
3. Read the chapter How to Use This Book. It'll give you a good idea of how to get started to get the most out of this book.
4. Lastly, collect your **FREE bonus tool kit** if you haven't already.

# HOW TO USE THIS BOOK

This is a playbook, which means you and I get to play. There are 8 valuable lessons. But just as I don't want doctors to approach each symptom or problem as a separate branch on a tree, I want to stress that these lessons are all connected. No matter in what order you approach this book, when you have read the whole thing, the connections of each chapter to each other will come through the pages. My favorite part of teaching in our programs is when I see people start to make these connections that they knew existed, but they finally put all the science together, and it makes total logical sense. Boom! Magic.

Use this book as a launching pad to open your understanding and approach to your health. It should make you question your doctor's and your paradigms. There should be ahas happening that will make you rethink your assumptions and theirs. This is a great thing.

I've learned from teaching thousands of people on the Transform System that people will come in thinking it's about one thing, and it becomes the gateway to learning about the beautiful tapestry piece by piece that's really what a root cause approach to health is all about.

**Always start with lesson number 1, which is to Lead with Curiosity.** That really sets the framework for the whole idea of play, learning, and expansion of your mind and your approach to your health. If you approach this book, your health, and your life with curiosity, everything changes. Sometimes, it's not what you approach but how you approach it that determines whether it's success versus failure. So, to approach the world through the lens of curiosity, you shall see it through the lens of the successful.

After the first lesson, **feel free to take a look at the lessons that appeal the most to you.** If you don't have time or you're someone who likes to read the end of the book, then here's a quick tip: read the action steps at the end of each chapter. The action steps behind each chapter are designed to be the most significant, most impactful first step to give someone a quick result or reward that would invite them to dig deeper.

Next, as you read this book, you're going to want to have **a highlighter ready and a pen.** Highlight anything you need; however, take notes in the **back of the book in the ACTION PLAN section.** Write down the page the insight came from, the main pearl or note you gleaned, and the action you will take. Then, when you've finished this book for the first time, you'll have a plan together to tackle some of your biggest health challenges.

I also invite you to go collect your bonus tool kit immediately. Besides being able to read the lessons, I would love to invite you to our training resources on our YouTube page, Facebook group, podcast, and in my programs, where I interact, play, teach, and laugh every

8 Out of the Box Ways to Transform Your Health
From Confusion to Confidence: The Playbook for Whole Body Wellness

day with real people like you who are eager to learn and transform their health. Lots of these episodes or sessions were recorded for you to search and learn from to deepen your understanding of the areas that affect you the most. The bonuses contain live training, videos, and frequently referenced resources that will create an experience for you. I don't just want you to read the book; I want you to consume it. I would love for you to get to know me and the people I've worked with better and how our stories and successes relate to you.

So have fun with it, start with curiosity, then dive into a lesson that interests you. Enjoy! And most importantly, I want to see and interact with you on my many social media lives, in workshops, and when speaking at events. I would love to meet you and sign your book. Connection is my highest value, and I want to set a collective intention of raising the bar and opportunities for connection with me and through me for you.

Stay connected and dive deeper into knowledge alongside me! Discover more through my speaking engagements, social media events, Facebook group activities, and live workshops. To enhance your journey, claim your bonuses and join our email list. Let's continue learning together!

**8 Out of the Box Ways to Transform Your Health**
From Confusion to Confidence: The Playbook for Whole Body Wellness

## Action Steps

1. Start with the first lesson about Leading with Curiosity. That's what's led me and so many others here.
2. After Leading with Curiosity, which sets the lens you look through, you can navigate through lessons based on your personal health curiosities and concerns.
3. If you're pressed for time or seeking swift insights, each lesson wraps up with actionable steps. The focus is to do those action items.
4. For those desiring a deep dive into specific topics, my YouTube channel offers a rich library of videos with real patient case studies, insights, and training.

5. Join our growing 92,229+ Facebook community, "Transform Your Health Naturally," to engage with the community, my team, and me directly. www.DrMaggieYu.com/Transform
6. Throughout each lesson, there are bonuses and tools that you can download and collect. We've collected them all here: www.8OutoftheBox.com/Bonus-Health

# LESSON 1:
## LEADING WITH CURIOSITY

### How Did We Get Here In Our Healthcare?

**The healthcare system is broken.** I had to come to the sad realization that our healthcare system inherently makes sick people sicker. The premise that this was a great system, creating great outcomes, and it was all altruistic about true healing, was all wrong. Something wasn't off. EVERYTHING was off. I wanted to scream. I wanted to cry. Most of all, I felt alone, hopeless, and sick while pretending to be the smiling doctor you loved to see. Until... I realized this was a system I could no longer participate in. It was not helping me and, in fact, was part of the problem.

Why does the current system fail? In the United States, the amount of money we spend on healthcare is outgrowing nearly every other area of spending. U.S. healthcare spending grew 2.7% in 2021, reaching 4.3 trillion or $12,914 per person per year. Healthcare spending accounted for 18.3% of the nation's Gross Domestic Product. Despite high healthcare spending, Americans have the lowest rates of physician visits, the lowest rate of practicing physicians, and some of the WORST outcomes.

According to CNN[1] the research shows that while Americans have a disproportionately high amount of healthcare spending, the outcomes compared to peer countries are one of the worst. The U.S. has one of the highest rates of deaths from avoidable or treatable causes. Americans live shorter, less healthy lives because our health system is not working. This isn't my opinion; this is a statistical fact, and you are living with the quality of your health every day. I was walking around sick, and ironically, I was just one of thousands of practicing doctors who were sick and delivering sick care. The outcomes of our healthcare system are terrible. Fact.

We've created a system that produces terrible health outcomes. We've also created a system that drives doctors out of the profession. Why are so many well-meaning doctors getting burned out and leaving in droves, never to return? We and they have invested so much into their training and learning. But the answer to why they're leaving lies in both what and how we are training our doctors.

There's a failure to train you and healthcare providers how to be curious. Our educational system is producing physicians and a healthcare system that is the opposite of what we need. We're training them to be robots on an assembly line. Being a product of the educational system and having educated and trained physicians, I know this system is a failure, and the results speak for themselves. I've been through the entire process of it. I was at UCLA, one of the top medical schools in the country. I was in a

[1] https://www.cnn.com/2023/01/31/health/us-health-care-spending-global-perspective/index.htm

wonderful family medicine residency. I practiced at the top medical groups and was one of the medical directors responsible for training other doctors in best practices. It wasn't until I was humbled by my own illnesses and mystery symptoms that I realized how I was educated and trained and was woefully unprepared for real-world vague, chronic, or a large number of symptoms involving multiple systems in an individual.

Every day, with each patient I encountered, I adhered to an ingrained system. I, along with other doctors, was trained to follow diagnostic checklists and algorithms meticulously. We'd funnel patients down predetermined paths based on their diagnosis and blood tests.

These routes, often resembling assembly lines, would direct them to further specialists, tests, or prescriptions. While this method might be efficient for many, it falls short for those with complex or unique symptoms, a category I eventually found myself in. Too often, our healthcare system shapes doctors to process patients quickly for the sake of efficiency rather than to heal. This assembly-line approach is a primary reason for physician burnout, as many enter the profession hoping to be healers, only to be caught in a cycle of rote memorization and protocol.

In my first ten years of practice, day in and day out was filled with an increasing number of patients who didn't fit the mold. I had to tell patient after patient that their lab or x-ray was normal and there wasn't a clear path I could send them down. We would offer these patients antidepressants and tell them to manage their stress or to work on losing weight. I was kind, and I cared, but there wasn't any prescription or additional test or referral I could do that would solve their problems. I was so frustrated at not being able to give so many of these people any answers or real help. Why? Those darn algorithms I was trained in.

The dictionary defines an algorithm as a process or set of rules to be followed in calculations or other problem-solving operations, especially by a computer. If a patient has heartburn, you must only prescribe antacids. If you have pain in an area, take an x-ray. If the antacids don't work or the x-ray doesn't show anything, the algorithm or questioning often stops or says to pass it on to someone else who has their next set of algorithms to go through. No wonder, as patients, we feel like we're not seen, heard, or dealt with as fully alive, sensitive, sentient human beings.

There's also medical liability associated with not following exact algorithms for doctors. Here's an example: a patient has high cholesterol, and she doesn't want to take a statin medication, so the doctor and patient agree that she will work on her cholesterol through a variety of other means. They agreed to retest her cholesterol and other cardiac tests to ensure the effectiveness of such treatments after a fixed period of time. However, the doctor receives a letter from the insurance that says, "Your patient with diabetes and cholesterol is not adhering to recommended guidelines. You must see the patient and document why or start this medication." Unfortunately, a physician cannot ignore this type of letter that they get tons of every day. This will require the physician to call or document in a visit with the patient that they're aware of this notice and deviation from a guideline and that the patient is declining the statin. This takes a ton of time and effort and is honestly a hassle. But in order to safely and legally navigate being a functional medicine doctor who supports other methods with medication being just one of the options and not the first and only option, there is a great deal of time, energy, and cost to documenting with defensive medicine. Doctors and patients are punished for exercising out-of-the-box thinking and practice. I've seen doctors fire patients who refuse to take a statin or other guideline-demanded treatments so they can mitigate legal risk.

It does not place enough emphasis on critical thinking; most crucially, it rarely nurtures the innate curiosity humans possess. Why didn't the antacid work? What else could it be? What's the real cause of this problem? Can this problem have multiple causes that an antacid may actually make worse? This is why common problems like heartburn typically go unsolved, and more and more health issues stack up due to underlying causes of heartburn that keep popping up later. We'll often hear someone ten years down the road say, "Wow, it started ten years ago as heartburn, and the antacid was prescribed, and we thought that was the end of that." Only now, this person has ulcerative colitis or ten years' worth of irritable bowel syndrome or neuropathy.

We are trained to treat people and medical conditions as computer problems or immediate-term mathematical equations to be solved. There's an inherent focus in our training only to treat the problem that's in front of us as quickly and with the least effort possible to be able to perform the same operation hundreds of times per week for our entire practicing lives. We were trained to be robotic operators to perform algorithms. This is a significant innate bias we have built into how we train physicians and how medical institutions operate.

Many doctors, including me, feel like we are waitresses serving a set menu. I was frustrated, overwhelmed by the complexity of many patients, and feeling helpless and hopeless. Like many of my colleagues, my original vision of how I would be a healer turned into a repeated nightmare of just being a cog in the machine. Even worse, after a decade of telling patients their labs were normal, and there was not much I could do, I became that sick patient nobody could explain. I felt totally alone with my symptoms and normal labs. I felt like a super special rare unicorn where nobody knew what was wrong with me. And I felt darn hopeless that anyone could help me. I became the overwhelmed, frustrated, and hopeless patient that I dreaded seeing the most.

At each step along my way, I started asking questions. The more symptoms I got, the more normal my labs were, the more questions came. These are questions I wasn't trained as a doctor to ask. I was more involved with things like how do I chart this, how do I get insurance to cover this or that, and how do I make it through the day being a cog. As I became a patient with more and more symptoms and got to more and more impasses, I had to learn a critical skill. I needed to be led by curiosity.

8 Out of the Box Ways to Transform Your Health
From Confusion to Confidence: The Playbook for Whole Body Wellness

**What is curiosity?** The dictionary defines it as having a strong desire to learn or know something. People with curiosity often don't need the information they're asking about. They're seeking answers to their questions for the sake of gaining knowledge. People who are curious often actively seek out challenges and new experiences to expand their minds.

Curiosity, as my core value, serves as a constant source of motivation for me to refine and perfect the art of asking increasingly insightful and meaningful questions. It's the driving force that propels me to dig deeper, explore the unknown, and uncover hidden layers of knowledge. With curiosity at my core, I recognize that the quality of my questions directly impacts the quality of the answers and solutions I can discover. Every question is an opportunity to expand my understanding, challenge assumptions, and foster meaningful connections with others. It's this insatiable thirst for knowledge and understanding that fuels my commitment to continuously honing the skill of asking better questions, ultimately leading to richer, more enlightening experiences and discoveries in both personal and professional realms. Curiosity, for me, is not just a value; it's a lifelong journey of intellectual growth and exploration. It is one of the core values of my business. Curiosity sets the stage for transformative growth and change. Being curious is a behavior that unlocks transformative results. The most important behavior of being curious is asking questions.

The quality of life is defined by the quality of the questions we ask. So, learn to ask better and better questions.

**8 Out of the Box Ways to Transform Your Health**
From Confusion to Confidence: The Playbook for Whole Body Wellness

It was very lonely for me not to have many colleagues to learn from or relate with in the early years. Over the years, it's become clear that many of my medical peers are grappling with personal health challenges, from chronic ailments to mental health struggles. The distressing statistics about suicides among healthcare professionals only deepened my unease. It made me wonder: Why are we turning to those most entrenched in the system, those facing similar struggles, for groundbreaking solutions?

I realized in my curiosity that you should explore the standard doctors and specialists for your problem. But if they're not curious, if they're not asking deeper questions, and if they don't foster and support your desire to do so, it is absolutely time to let curiosity lead you elsewhere. There are so many other people and other tools that your questions will lead you to!

## What Does a Curiosity-Led Adventure Look Like with One Common Symptom?

Let's consider a common issue that you, or someone close to you, may have faced - constipation, the struggle to have regular bowel movements. The current healthcare system can be likened to this condition. We introduce less-than-ideal components into our systems, operate with a less-than-optimal digestion mechanism, and consequently fail to absorb essential nutrients or health advantages. We accumulate issues, misdiagnoses, and ailments.

Consequently, our inability to regularly cleanse our systems results in a repetitive cycle of toxin retention. In essence, the contemporary healthcare system is plagued with inefficiencies, characterized by its incapacity to discard waste and elevate its efficacy.

But what if we viewed constipation from a perspective of curiosity? Firstly, it's crucial to respect our symptoms. These symptoms act as signals, a mode of communication from our body to our consciousness. Our digestive system, albeit voiceless, is constantly trying to convey messages. Embracing curiosity means recognizing and valuing these signs. Upon experiencing constipation, probe your body with questions like:

- Bowels, what are you silently trying to tell me?
- If you had a voice, what would it say?
- What burdens am I clinging to that no longer serves me?
- Which negative influences in my life remain unaddressed and keep circulating?
- Are there specific muscular tensions I'm only now becoming conscious of?
- How does this muscular tension show up elsewhere?
- What emotion primarily surfaces when I experience constipation?
- When did this symptom first appear? Can I recall its inception?
- Do I prioritize my body's needs and signals?
- Am I being too rigid with my body, imposing my schedules on it?
- What's my mindset when attempting to poop?

**8 Out of the Box Ways to Transform Your Health**
From Confusion to Confidence: The Playbook for Whole Body Wellness

- Does pooping induce pain, perhaps suggesting an aversion to discomfort?
- Are there emotions linked to this act that I wish to evade, and where else do they reflect in my life?
- In what other facets of my life do I feel trapped or stagnated?
- How is my thought process hindered?
- Are there aspects of this issue I might be overlooking?
- Have I asked someone else if there is something they see that I don't?
- Who else can offer valuable insights on this?
- Where can I find reliable, tailored information pertinent to my unique situation, grounded in science?
- How long will I tolerate this issue before I try a different approach to get a different outcome?
- Could this issue be a manifestation of another underlying problem?
- Are there genetic predispositions, ancestral health patterns, past surgeries, or personal medical records linked to this issue?
- Who has successfully overcome constipation, and how?
- Who do I need to speak to that could offer new perspectives or solutions I haven't yet encountered?
- How can I objectively monitor improvements to track my progress?

Engaging with such thought-provoking questions can easily lead us down a rabbit hole of discovery. Remember, the quality of your life often hinges on the quality of the questions you ask. Can you envision how this curiosity-driven approach can introduce you to fresh perspectives, knowledge, remedies, strategies, and outcomes? From my personal journey, I've found that refining the art of questions not only amplified my knowledge but also significantly enhanced my health outcomes.

## The Cheat Sheet on Curiosity Lead Questions

The five W's of curiosity-based questions:

- Who?
- What?
- Where?
- Why?
- When?

In a provider or encounter with anyone about health, it looks like:

- Who got different results in this situation?
- What did they do differently that helped?
- Where did this person get help? Where did they learn this?
- Why did they seek this method?
- When did you see this person or hear about them? When in their treatment did you decide to take this route?

Here are examples of additional "what" questions:
- What haven't we tried?
- What is something I'm possibly not seeing about this situation?
- What else would you do?
- What do you think is really causing this problem?
- What's something new you've learned about this that was fascinating?

My favorite question always to add to this isn't a question at all; it's the statement: tell me more.

With each of your symptoms, or in preparation for your medical visits, a couple of the questions above can open up a world of new possibilities and connections.

These types of questions have helped me quickly identify the curious and intelligent people I want to connect with. These people then always connected me with information or people that led and elevated me to a life I never imagined.

## My Own Journey Through Pain Led by Curiosity as a Case Study

**The chiropractors who expanded the landscape.** Chronic pain gripped my life and has been my constant companion since the age of 23, with a disc herniation in my low back. From there, I developed postpartum fibromyalgia, shoulder and wrist pain, TMJ, neck pain from a car accident, multiple neck surgeries, a broken foot requiring more surgery, and painful nerve pain on my face and neck with neuropathy.

No medicine, not one doctor, not one medication, and not one surgery ended any of the pain. Each added to the last so that pain became the constant language of my own body. Besides all the conventional traditional medical care I received that didn't work, I had to ask more questions and drive myself to new doctors, new supplements, new medications, new procedures, and new modalities. I couldn't live with the unacceptable result of living with this level of escalating pain every day.

My quest for answers took me to many chiropractors, where I was met with temporary relief. However, it was through my many questions and connections with them that I was eventually introduced to a specialized field of chiropractic care, the National Upper Cervical Chiropractic Association (NUCCA). There are subspecialties in chiropractics. Did you know that? These specialists focus on adjusting the upper neck area, the first several vertebrates, which are difficult or impossible for regular chiropractors to adjust. Here, I began to explore the potential connection between my severe jaw, mental health issues, and my pain, which appeared to stem from higher up in my neck. This journey opened my eyes to the diverse world of chiropractic care and its various specializations. Ask questions so you understand who in the area of health you need answers for.

The big takeaway: learn as much as you can about the profession of the professionals you're seeing. In the health problem you're tackling, do you understand the hierarchy, the subspeciality, or the outliers that are dealing with it? Ask a ton of questions, find out who your rheumatologist sees when they're sick. Who's the endocrinologist to the endocrinologists? Who's on social media and YouTube that's teaching something different or contrarian to everyone else? Learn the landscape.

**MELT Method: The fascia connection.** Another pivotal moment in my search for relief was my encounter with Amanda, a client who also happened to be a MELT movement instructor. She asked a question that would light the path in a different direction. I asked her, "What are you seeing that I'm not seeing? She answered with yet another question, "What if this is not related to bone, nerves, or muscle but to your fascia?" This question challenged the medical knowledge I had acquired, which had neglected the significance of fascia. With her guidance, I ventured into the world of the MELT Method, finding profound relief from my chronic neck pain.

To start with, what is fascia? It is a thin casing of connective tissue that surrounds and holds every organ, blood vessel, bone, nerve fiber, and muscle in place. The tissue does more than provide internal structure; fascia has nerves that make it almost as sensitive as skin. When stressed, it tightens up. As you can see, it's not just a thin white sheet of fibers that covers each organ; it's got nerves, it's got water molecules, calcium crystals, nerves, and it is packed full of immune cells and tissue memory. Fascia holds powerful stimulation and balance to our nervous system, and it plays a role in the storage and release of hormones. Fascia communicates throughout the body and has anatomical planes and layers none of us doctors have ever learned about. We don't get it. Like I said, doctors think it's just something we cut through that's in the way.

I met Sue Hitzmann, the brilliant mind behind the MELT Method. Her humility, curiosity, and spiritual depth have enriched my understanding of how fascia influences pain, hormone imbalances, and digestive concerns. This profound knowledge is why the MELT Method is central to our programs and why educating about fascia is essential. I can't imagine how my journey with chronic pain and the struggles of thousands of others could've ended without the experience and training of experts like Sue or other bodyworkers.

The big takeaway: Move, no matter what, keep moving. Find a form of movement that you can do. Learn from movement experts who have had to overcome their own health issues. YouTube their videos and try out as many different modalities as it takes for you to find something that you enjoy that has an impact. Check out MELT Method on YouTube. Success leaves clues; the technique and tools have helped thousands just in our programs alone.

**Linda Caravia LMT: A Unique Approach to Massage.** The introduction of Linda Caravia, a licensed massage therapist (LMT) specializing in Sarga massage, further enriched my understanding of the body. Her innovative approach involved using her feet to apply friction and pressure to reach deep layers of fascia. Unlike previous massage therapists, Linda's inquisitive nature and personalized approach prompted an in-depth exploration of my anatomy. She consistently asked questions and shared insights that surpassed my medical education. Her expertise reshaped my perspective on anatomy and deepened my appreciation for the power of curiosity.

The big takeaway? Find your tribe. Curiosity out to the universe brings it back. In my search for providers to help me with pain, Linda taught me the most about how to find someone to geek out with. Find people who are geeking out on your problem and join them!

**Dr. Bryan Baisinger: The Fascia Visionary,** a chiropractor with a passion for fascia work, provided the next breakthrough in my healing journey. His unconventional methods and extensive knowledge of the body were unlike anything I had encountered in traditional chiropractic care. Under his guidance, I uncovered the influence of fascia in areas I had never considered, from my chest and breast to my pelvis. His approach extended beyond bone adjustments, focusing on the release of fascia and scar tissue, leading to transformative results.

The big takeaway: the best teachers are outliers. Find the people who have gone above and beyond their professional bubble. Bryan is a chiropractor whose main goal in life is not to adjust your bones. He's the only chiropractor who has worked on soft tissue for a long time. He's the only one who spends a long time teaching his patients his deep knowledge. He gets totally out-of-the-box results. He's spending most of his time teaching his team and his patients, not cracking and leaving. Everything about him is an outlier. Find the outliers who are solving your problem in a totally different way. Learn from them, see them, pay them, thank them. It takes a lot of grit to be the outlier in your profession. (Trust me, I know.)

**The emotional release and trauma connection.** As my journey continued, the pelvic floor release work led me straight into trauma-release work, unearthing buried emotions and memories hidden within my fascial tissue. Pain, vibrations, temperatures, and sensations emerged as a language spoken by the body, providing valuable data points. Therapeutic techniques such as Somatic therapy, Eye Movement Desensitization Reprocessing therapy (EMDR), Internal Family Systems Therapy (IFS), and Polyvagal theory bridged the gap between experiences, thoughts, and physical sensations. The journey through trauma-release work not only healed my body but also transformed my thoughts to be present. I am no longer trapped by my memories and stories from the past with my pain. The journey continues today. In order to leave pain behind, I had to release the pain I felt inside.

The big takeaway: your body has memory, and it is speaking to you. When are you going to listen, when are you going to interpret, and when are you going to trust it? It's time.

## Conclusion

I'm truly thankful for the opportunity to share my pain journey. Every piece that's hurt led me to new questions, new answers, new providers. It's led me to many out-of-the-box providers and nonmedical providers alike. I have found answers outside, and inside myself I never anticipated.

Lead with childlike, open, and playful curiosity instead of an inquisition. I've asked these questions to myself or have been asked by others, and some of these answers can only come out in a safe, open, and learning environment. These teachers and mentors I've shared with you have inspired me to share my story, my insights, and my solutions.

This lesson answers the many 5 Ws of how I ended my pain journey—the who, what, why, where, and when. So, in your health journey, start asking everyone these questions. Make sure you also add to the questions the statement, tell me more. It will be the beginning of a beautiful journey. Oh, the places you'll go.

If you are curious to learn more about ways to lead with your mind and how to develop tools to be aware of your own thoughts. Be sure to read the lesson **Mindset to Mind Growth.**

## Action Steps

I've provided you with some curiosity-based questions and room to journal. Take each question and give yourself a minute at least before you start to write an answer. If you need more room to write your answers, feel free to stay with a particular question and add additional pieces of paper for an extended answer.

Each question is a process I want you to do so that you begin to lead this problem with curiosity.

**List of curiosity-based questions to ask yourself to understand your health in more depth. These are led by the 5 Ws: who, what, where, when, why.**

- What is one of my current medical problems? Is that really the problem?

..................................................................................................
..................................................................................................
..................................................................................................
..................................................................................................
..................................................................................................
..................................................................................................

- Who have I been told about that I haven't explored, and why? Is there resistance from me?

..................................................................................................
..................................................................................................
..................................................................................................
..................................................................................................
..................................................................................................
..................................................................................................

- What haven't I done, what haven't I tried? Why not?

..................................................................................
..................................................................................
..................................................................................
..................................................................................
..................................................................................
..................................................................................

- What is something I'm possibly not seeing about this situation? Ask as many people around you as possible this same question. You can't always see what they see.

..................................................................................
..................................................................................
..................................................................................
..................................................................................
..................................................................................
..................................................................................

- Where in my body, if I had to point, would be the actual cause of this problem?

..................................................................................
..................................................................................
..................................................................................
..................................................................................
..................................................................................
..................................................................................

- What emotion do I feel when I point to the body part that's sick? When did I first feel that?

..................................................................................................
..................................................................................................
..................................................................................................
..................................................................................................
..................................................................................................
..................................................................................................

- If I could do something different or better in this situation, what would that be? Ask everyone this question about any situation.

..................................................................................................
..................................................................................................
..................................................................................................
..................................................................................................
..................................................................................................
..................................................................................................

- What do I think is really causing this problem? Ask every provider this question.

..................................................................................................
..................................................................................................
..................................................................................................
..................................................................................................
..................................................................................................
..................................................................................................

- What's something new I've learned on this topic that's fascinating? (Ask each of your providers this very same question about this issue.)

..................................................................................
..................................................................................
..................................................................................
..................................................................................
..................................................................................
..................................................................................

- Do I know anyone who has been able to get different results on this? Who?

..................................................................................
..................................................................................
..................................................................................
..................................................................................
..................................................................................
..................................................................................

- Another person who's been successful at solving this problem, what are they doing differently? When is the symptom or diagnosis the best time to consider this idea or treatment? The right thing at the wrong time isn't the right thing.

..................................................................................
..................................................................................
..................................................................................
..................................................................................
..................................................................................
..................................................................................

- When and what is the first step I need to take?

..................................................................................................
..................................................................................................
..................................................................................................
..................................................................................................
..................................................................................................

**Bonus:** Take the problem, symptom, or diagnosis you have, visit my YouTube channel, and put that symptom or problem into the search. Watch one to two stories of someone else who's been successful with turning this problem around, take notes, what are they doing you're not? Answer the questions above as you watch their path to success. Success leaves clues; look at someone who's successfully solved your problem, and write down all the answers to the questions above as you listen to them share their experience. That's your roadmap.

# LESSON 2:
## DIGESTION - THE FIRST DOMINO

*Thomas is a 46-year-old rowing enthusiast and instructor living in Boston. However, he has struggled with knee and hip pain for the past three years, limiting how long he can row. Despite seeing an orthopedist, no cause has been identified for his pain, and his x-rays appeared normal. Thomas has also gained 20 pounds and has had a major depressive episode.*

*On top of all of this, Thomas has been experiencing indigestion for several years. He had pain and discomfort after he ate. At the same time, he was previously prescribed medication to reduce stomach acid. He had short-term relief, but the symptoms have returned. He stayed on the heartburn medication, but then, a few months later, he felt extended periods of fullness and abdominal bloating after eating. Thomas has also noticed that his eczema has worsened, and he has developed dandruff on his scalp.*

*When I first met Thomas, he was experiencing a whole range of health issues. Over the past three years, he had seen his primary care doctor, a gastroenterologist, several dermatologists, and an orthopedist. He also saw an acupuncturist and energy healer and was still struggling to get results. His wife had urged him to seek counseling for his depressed mood. Thomas's health was impacting his ability to be active, his mood, his relationship with his wife, and now impacting his work as an analyst at a bank. As frustrated as he was, his wife was the one who initially reached out to us. She was into healthy eating and natural forms of medicine and knew that there had to be other options than more medications and referrals.*

*When we first discussed his case, there were many clues in his story pointing to digestive issues, which impacted many other parts of his body and mental health. It was a very different starting place than they or his doctors had thought. As both him and his wife learned about all the steps in digestion, they began to realize just how much their doctors and they had missed. No one had considered his myriad of symptoms linked or some key points in his family's history.*

*Not surprisingly, he found that his indigestion and abdominal pain stopped within a few weeks. Within a short time after that, he stopped taking his omeprazole, an acid-suppressing medication. Additionally, his left foot pain disappeared, and two months later, he reported no knee pain. Most shockingly, his eczema and dandruff had completely cleared up.*

*When I met with Thomas recently in one of our virtual group meetings, he had lost 14 pounds and had resumed rowing. He had even taken up karate and was enjoying a new hobby of riding motorcycles with his brother-in-law. Overall, Thomas was feeling much healthier and happier. His wife Sandy celebrated a win for the both of them. She had lifelong constipation that ended, and she noticed that the rosacea redness on her face and cheeks was gone. Their health journeys' turnarounds all started with addressing his digestive issues.*

## What's Wrong with the Current Approach?

Thomas's case is typical of so many with chronic health symptoms. Many of you reading this book and the people we work with report some sort of digestion-related symptom in their history or in their family history. Highlight the symptoms below that you experience that could point you to your own digestion problems.

These are clues in Thomas's story that your doctor may not make the connection to digestion:

- Knee and hip pain
- Weight gain
- Depression
- Indigestion
- Fullness after eating
- Bloating
- Eczema
- Dandruff

In this chapter, we'll be able to link every one of his symptoms and help you understand why they are clues not to be missed, pointing directly at the real problem: there were steps in his digestion that are not working correctly.

Why is there no attention paid to digestion as the cause of so many symptoms? The issue here is that medical doctors need more formal training in digestion. In all my years of medical school, family medicine residency training, and even going through gastrointestinal rotations learning from those doctors, I had never received any in-depth training on digestion. My colleagues from all the other medical schools had the same experience. Primary care doctors and gastroenterologists are trained on the symptoms; here are the tests to perform, if any, and here's what to prescribe. This is a classic example of how doctors are trained on algorithms and flow charts of what steps to take, like a warehouse sorting facility. When the doctors you go to see are there to sort or give you a test or treatment only, there's simply no opportunity to dig deeper. There's neither time, capacity, nor the curiosity to do so. We were just taught that if someone has a symptom like heartburn, prescribe a medicine like omeprazole to shut off stomach acid.

This was and still is the standard of care. Turn off parts of their digestion as a long-term strategy, until years later, problems relating to the long-term prescription of acid-blocking medications reveal the long-term effects of shutting off parts of digestion.

Shutting it off didn't work? Okay, let's remove it.

Gallbladder issues are common, and it's likely you know someone who's had theirs removed, or perhaps you have. At its core, the root cause of gallbladder problems often stems from issues related to digesting fats: producing bile, storing bile acids, and releasing them effectively for fat breakdown. Disruptions in this cycle can lead to pain in the gallbladder or liver region. Over time, this can result in the accumulation of grit or even stones in the gallbladder, affecting its function. But instead of addressing the early warning signs and underlying issues with fat digestion, conventional medicine often only intervenes when there's a critical problem—like large gallstones causing obstructions, intense pain, or even infections.

This reactive approach, focusing on immediate emergencies rather than preventing them, often results in the removal of the gallbladder, a crucial organ for digestion. The real tragedy is that many early symptoms of poor fat digestion go unnoticed, partly due to the lack of adequate tools and training available to practitioners.

However, removing the organ responsible for most of the fat digestion in the body only exacerbates the issue. Without the gallbladder, the body has little to no fat digestion capabilities. In fact, the downstream effects of being unable to digest and absorb fat became a much bigger problem. Proper fat digestion is essential for the body's holistic well-being, impacting everything from our immediate health to our lifespan. Symptoms associated with poor fat digestion include some ubiquitous ones, from neuropathy, hormone imbalances, and eczema to chronic pain, brain fog, fatigue, and depression. While these connections will be further unpacked later, an immediate emphasis should be on our diets. After all, doesn't the very essence of what we consume demand our utmost attention?

Do natural-leaning doctors have the answers, then? Some naturopathic or functional practitioners recommend supplements to aid digestion. While they might recognize symptoms like bloating as an indicator of digestive issues and suggest remedies accordingly, there often needs to be a link in their approach. For instance, while a naturopathic physician might understand the bloating, they may not connect this broken step in digestion to other symptoms like depression, eczema, or chronic pain, as we saw in Thomas's case. They also wouldn't necessarily know how to manage Thomas's other medical diagnosis or medications.

A combined approach is explained in this chapter, so while learning about the root causes around digestion, you begin to see how they cause and impact your medical diagnosis and medications. This chapter aims to unravel and highlight these often-overlooked connections between digestion and broader health concerns for doctors and patients alike. To help medical professionals, holistic providers, and the general public gain access to learn how to combine the tools from multiple approaches, I had to figure out a way to teach and integrate both to everyone. To bridge this chasm, I had to create health learning programs that combined traditional medicine and holistic medicine through a mix of video sessions, reading materials, worksheets, and interactive troubleshooting sessions with providers who have trained on both sides of the fence. We also lean heavily into live, experiential teaching, using real stories and results to underscore lessons. These personal narratives act as a potent reinforcement, equipping individuals with the knowledge and confidence to address and navigate any health issues, including digestive issues. I built the learning on people participating in small learning circles led by mentors, and this created communities and support.

This lesson is a quick, laser-focused, and in-depth lesson to help you connect the dots between this one problem and the rest of your health symptoms. Next stop, let's talk about food.

# Food Matters, Digestion Matters More

Let me paint a picture for you. You're opening a bakery. You focus on sourcing the best ingredients, talk to vendors, test recipes at home, and try eating at all these other bakeries, focusing on your recipes and your ingredients in great depth. That makes sense. Meanwhile, your bakery has an oven that doesn't reach or keep the temperature well. Your main mixer has a blown fuse and isn't working. What about a vacuum sealer that's broken, so you can't seal the items you bake? Can you produce the results you want? Can you open and can you serve customers? The answer is clearly no.

While food or the ingredients going into the bakery clearly matters. The most crucial first step is to make sure you have a properly functioning kitchen where every step of the baking process is working perfectly.

Why focus on the best vanilla from Madagascar when you can't even use it in a recipe because the mixer is down? The kitchen is your digestive tract. Every single step involves a specific part of your body. Each step has a specific product and function. And every step is critical to the outcome. You have to get the system the food is processed in to be optimal to get the best-tasting, consistent, and nutrient-dense food you're trying to create. This is why I am making the statement: order matters; get the digestion right first!

*Brenda was down to just seven foods. That's total. For years, she had swollen lips and tingling tongues to food. When she ate, she developed a stomach ache with immediate diarrhea. She had unexplained hives, which were itchy on her skin. She had chronic sinus fullness and asthma, requiring daily use of a steroid inhaler. She wasn't the only one; both her children had unexplained allergic reactions. She's been so traumatized by these unexplained food reactions that it's made it difficult for her to travel or even plan her day. The problem is, no matter how much food she eliminated, her reactions only reduced nominally. Why?*

**Digestion reduces allergens.** Most people and even functional medicine providers dealing with chronic symptoms focus on food. It's an easy focus because many people have allergic or other acute reactions to food. Most people do have bad eating habits, and that definitely needs to change. Unfortunately, by focusing on food first, we go to great lengths and expenses to decrease our symptoms. Still, the food restrictions or changes don't often create the tangible or measurable responses we had hoped for, as the food is not getting properly digested. One example is people with allergic reactions to food. You'd think eliminating more and more that'd produce quick results, right? Yet it doesn't.

**Digestion is our body's mechanism to break down food into smaller molecules,** small enough to be absorbed and utilized. This intricate process, when functioning correctly, ensures that allergenic particles in our food are broken down into even smaller components. Although the body might still identify them as allergens, the reduced size and load mean fewer histamines and inflammatory reactions in the gut.

Thus, by leveraging our digestive system's capabilities, we can mitigate the allergic responses to certain foods.

Enhanced digestion has the potential to alleviate conditions like IBS, allergies, mast cell activation disorder, or histamine intolerance. By simplifying allergenic particles into more digestible fragments, one can not only achieve better digestion but also reduce the adverse symptoms associated with food allergies.

*Consider Dina, a stark representation of the consequences of impaired digestion. Suffering from Postural Orthostatic Tachycardia Syndrome (POTS) and Mast Cell Activation Syndrome (MCAS), Dina faced severe malabsorption issues. The absence of vital stomach acid and pancreatic enzymes rendered her unable to digest her food. Even the multitude of supplements she consumed proved futile as her body struggled to break them down and absorb their benefits. It's little surprise she weighed a mere ninety-six pounds and battled weight gain. Moreover, undigested food, toxins, and allergens in her system triggered a myriad of reactions, leading to erratic and fluctuating symptoms throughout the day.*

**Digestion decreases infection in your body.** There are several reasons why infections are rampant in our intestines, such as a lack of intestinal bacteria diversity, resulting in fewer good bacteria to perform essential functions in our body. When there are fewer good bacteria in our gut to perform basic and advanced functions, such as immunity, the ability of our gut to protect us from infection decreases. As a result, we are finding more and more infections in our intestines. The role of underlying infections is covered in another lesson in depth.

**Poor digestion of food affects the nutrients your large intestinal bacteria get.** Each digestion step is a line of defense for your gut. The good bacteria play a pivotal role in hormone production and breakdown. Any disruption in the preceding digestive steps jeopardizes our hormonal balance, culminating in the final fermentation step: a process heavily dependent on the presence and nourishment of good bacteria. When these bacteria aren't properly nurtured, it leads to an accumulation of toxins, excessive hormones, and potential infections. Some individuals struggle with weight loss due to an imbalance in these beneficial bacteria, often stemming from earlier, broken digestive steps. Given these cascading impacts, it's clear why prioritizing digestion is crucial.

## Understanding the Steps in Digestion

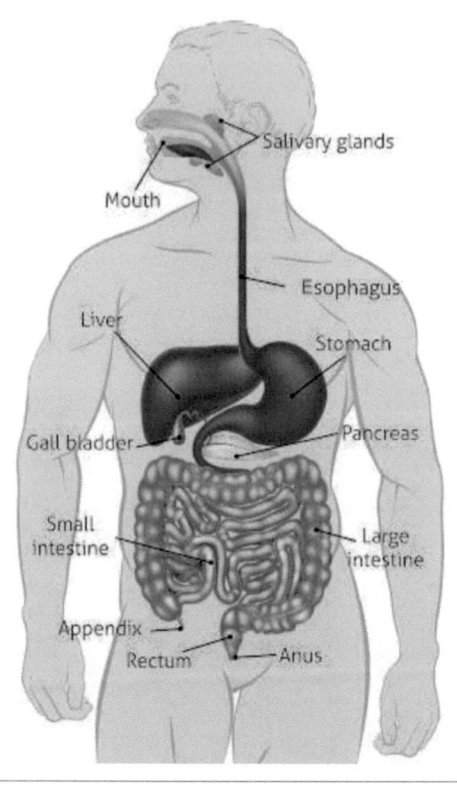

**Hydration** is crucial for proper digestion and biochemical processes throughout the body. This is why one of the first things we do when working with clients is our 10-Day Hydration Challenge, which helps people calculate the adequate amount of water they need. Adequate hydration is essential because it lubricates food.

Drinking water throughout the day dilutes your body's fluids, which is why proper hydration is crucial. Drinking water while eating helps dilute the food, making it easier to break it down into smaller molecules for better digestion and decreased allergen load.

**Action step:** Drink a full glass of water before eating. Sip water throughout your meal to aid dilution and digestion.

**Mastication** is simply the act of chewing your food. Surprisingly, many people rush through their meals without adequately chewing their food. Unfortunately, many people simply gulp down their food without taking the time to chew it properly.

I recall a story about my sister, who was in her late 30s when her husband pointed out that she never properly chewed rice. She would simply put it in her mouth and swallow it whole. When he brought this to her, she replied, "Isn't that what everybody does?" Unfortunately, this is a common problem. When we fail to chew our food properly, we're doing our bodies a disservice. Proper chewing helps to break down food into smaller particles, which aids in digestion and absorption. If we swallow large chunks of food, we ask our digestive system to work harder downstream to break it down into smaller pieces. This can be challenging for the body and lead to digestive issues.

Notice when you eat next time, how many times you chew your food, and how much you don't chew and swallow in big chunks.

**Action step:** Chew each bite of your food at least ten times before swallowing it.

**Stomach acid is the hero, not the villain.** Acid breaks down food into smaller particles and sanitizes against infection. Unfortunately, many people have impaired stomach acid production genetically or due to factors such as infection, alcohol consumption, or certain medications. As a result, symptoms of low stomach acid, such as bloating and difficulty digesting meat, are common.

Bloating is the number one symptom of low stomach acid and can be worse for people who eat meat since it requires more stomach acid to break down and absorb. It's important to note that low stomach acid can cause various diseases and symptoms, including difficulties tolerating foods and vitamin and nutrient deficiencies. However, doctors are not trained to recognize these symptoms.

So, the question arises, "What can help improve stomach acid?" Unfortunately, if it's genetic, there's not much you can do but start taking stomach acid. That's why, for us, a multi-phasic digestive enzyme like DIGEST-IT is a game-changer for so many people.

Thomas's case is a classic example of low stomach acid. He presented with heartburn and indigestion. This symptom is classically misdiagnosed as having too much stomach acid. Conventional doctors will then prescribe him omeprazole to shut it down. Long term, he did not improve on the medication and then developed prolonged fullness with bloating, both of which are classic symptoms of low stomach acid.

Remember Brenda, who was down to seven foods, and eliminating more foods didn't help her reactions to food? Within two weeks of her being on DIGEST-IT, her symptoms were gone. She had low stomach acid and couldn't digest her food or handle the allergens in her food. They needed stomach acid to break down in her stomach. This is how powerful understanding digestion is. Because for her and many others, the symptoms got so severe that they caused pain, insomnia, diarrhea, rashes, and social anxiety. You get traumatized, being afraid of food because it can be eating anything. So it's not even like a specific food you can avoid when you have a digestion problem. It wasn't so much an ingredient in a bakery problem; it was the oven or the mixer that needed to be fixed.

**DIGEST-IT** is a multi-phasic digestive enzyme designed to provide stomach acid, protein digestion, and ox bile to aid in fat digestion problems.

- DIGEST-IT also includes the enzyme lactase, which

helps break down the dairy sugar lactose.
- The use of DIGEST-IT before meals may be helpful for patients who experience gas and bloating after eating, occasional constipation, or a feeling of fullness after eating only a small quantity of food.
- We recommend starting one with small meals and two capsules with big meals.

Food trauma is real. Brenda was afraid to put any food in her mouth. She was traumatized every time she ate, but we all have to eat every day. We wonder why so many people have eating disorders. Just digestive problems alone, unrecognized and untreated, routinely and randomly cause adverse effects with food consumption. We then look at little kids to adults and can understand why so many have food aversions and others have social anxiety around food.

Brenda's problem was solved in many different ways. However, the first and most important step for her and Thomas was to understand the steps in digestion. By addressing her low stomach acid by taking a product that contains stomach acid, she had quick results that gave her confidence that she was on the right path. By the way, she's now up to over 50 foods, has no rashes, and is back full-time in her therapist practice.

**Action step:** Try a multi-phasic digestive product like DIGEST-IT that contains stomach acid to see if it decreases symptoms of bloating, poor meat digestion, or constipation.

**Pancreas:** the masked Avenger. The pancreas is a

powerful organ that creates hormones, produces insulin, and many digestive enzymes like amylase, lipase, and many other digestive factors like acids, chemicals, and salts, all used in the digestive process. The pancreas is an organ often ignored. Doctors frequently only associate it with insulin hormone production and diabetes. Many people, including me, have poor pancreatic digestive function. Advanced stool tests can help measure some of these products of pancreatic digestion. So, I have data to show that a lot of people with certain types of diseases have impaired pancreatic digestion of food. It sits right after your stomach towards your small intestine and secretes enzymes and digestive factors that can digest carbohydrates, proteins, and even some fat.

When you don't have good gallbladder or pancreatic digestion, food from your stomach can slowly empty into your small intestine because the capacity to digest is decreased or slowed. Recall that Thomas felt full after eating for hours. Besides low stomach acid, he also had low pancreatic enzymes based on his symptoms, later verified with other testing.

You can experience symptoms where you feel full, or food feels like it's sitting there for a long time. It can cause fullness, pain, and discomfort. Poor pancreas digestion can also affect your ability to digest certain sugars or carbohydrates, which can cause gas and stomach aches after eating. You may think you're allergic to certain foods, but you may have a digestive problem that doesn't digest those sugars.

This is a significant problem to understand: the pancreas

plays a big role in digesting many different macro and micronutrients that come through your intestine. It's often difficult to diagnose through standard testing for pancreatic enzyme deficiency. The easiest way to see if you have this problem is to take pancreatic enzyme support to see if it helps.

**Action step:** take a multi-phasic digestive product like DIGEST-IT that includes pancreatic enzyme support to aid in the digestion of protein, carbohydrates, and fats.

**The liver** has a critical role in digestion and has many other functions. People often think of it only as a detoxification organ. The liver plays a significant role in making hormones and breaking down hormones and toxins. In fat digestion, the liver creates bile acids and salts, which go into the gallbladder and impact fat digestion. Unfortunately, we are facing a crisis with people experiencing decreased liver function due to non-alcoholic fatty liver disease. Blood sugar problems often cause fatty liver.

An impaired fatty liver will impair digestion. The role of the liver in blood sugar balance, hormone synthesis, and breakdown are discussed elsewhere.

The liver's role in the breakdown of toxins from infection is also another reason for fatty liver and impaired liver digestion of fats.

Let's add another layer to this: issues with fat digestion can also contribute to neuropathy. Yes, it's a lot to digest (no pun intended). You see, your nerves rely on healthy fats for optimal function. Problems absorbing essential omega-3 fats can trigger nerve problems, including dementia and impaired brain function. So, supplementing with high-quality omega-3, like our PRO-OMEGA 1000, can be a powerful strategy for tackling neuropathy. Action step for neuropathy: take PRO-OMEGA 1000 or a high-quality omega-3 at doses needed to combat neuropathy, about 3000 mg/day.

**PRO-OMEGA 1000** contains high levels of omega-3s with eicosapentaenoic acid (EPA), which has been clinically shown to be an incredible anti-inflammatory for pain, decreasing autoimmune symptoms, mood support, and immune support. I take 3000-4000 mg daily!

- **What it does:** Supports healthy hormones, heart, head, and hair, helpful for hormone balance and inflammation.
- **How it helps:** Omega 3 fatty acids are an essential nutrient that our body requires to maintain optimum health. Our Standard American Diet does not contain enough of these essential fatty acids, and they are foundational to improving heart and brain health and lowering inflammation in the body.
- Our bodies can make a small amount of eicosapentaenoic acid (EPA) and docosahexaenoic acid (DHA), but consuming sources of omega-3 fatty acids from diet or supplementation is vital for the maintenance of good health.
- **Directions:** Take one in the morning and two before bed.

**Action step:** Balance blood sugars by bookending the

day; you can read more on this in **Blood Sugar Mastery.** Consider fatty liver support supplementation such as LIVER LOVE to aid in the recovery from fatty liver and to optimize liver function. Add essential omega-3 fatty acids to your diet, suggested by food rich in omega-3s, or take PRO-OMEGA 1000 at three tablets per day.

**The gallbladder** helps the liver break down fat. When fat enters the small intestine, digestive hormones send signals to the gallbladder, which stores bile acid from the liver, to contract. These bile acids enter the small intestine to help sequester, meaning surround, the fat molecules into smaller and smaller molecules so that they can be digested and absorbed. Despite its importance, gallbladder removal surgeries are one of the most common surgeries worldwide. How many of you have had your gallbladder removed? How many of you can tell when you eat fatty foods; it just sits there? How many of your doctors have ignored these complaints?

We find that when there is an underlying fat digestion problem, whether it's from the liver or gallbladder, doctors often fail to address the root cause.
Instead of asking, "How can we help the liver or gallbladder?" They wait until the gallbladder is clogged with stones or infected, causing pain, at which point surgical removal is often the only solution. The surgery itself removes a vital organ for digesting fat.

After the surgery, no explanation or recommendations

are made for the patient to take digestive supports or Ox Bile supplements to digest their fats.

Symptoms of gallbladder or fat digestion problems include floating, greasy, or smelly stools due to undigested fat moving to the large intestine and abdominal pain after eating a fatty meal caused by the gallbladder's struggle to contract around stones or sand. If you experience these symptoms, addressing the underlying digestion issue is crucial. If you've had your gallbladder removed, you must, even more importantly, manage your lack of fat digestion long-term.

Poor fat digestion leads to immediate symptoms, as we've discussed. Still, downstream, if you don't absorb fat, you don't get essential fatty acids and omegas necessary to make hormones or heal nerves. No wonder so many people with neuropathy or chronic pain are on low-fat diets. Or they're eating fat, but it's not getting absorbed, which is another missed opportunity to help pain or mental health problems that involve brain and nerve cells.

**Action step:** Take DIGEST-IT, which contains Ox Bile to aid in fat digestion. If you do not have a gallbladder or your ability to digest fat is low, you may have to add additional Ox Bile to DIGEST-IT to fat-heavy meals. Make sure you're still eating fat!

**Fermentation** is the final step in digestion, and it relies on the good bacteria in your gut. When prebiotics from fiber are fermented, they create short-chain fatty acids that have many beneficial effects, including helping break down hormones and detoxifying the body. Good bacterial fermentation is essential for these processes, making good bacteria a vital component of the final step in digestion. We will dive into this process further in our Microbiome chapter. The big takeaway is that any step that's broken before it will cause this final step of fermentation not to occur correctly.

The immediate problem for those who don't ferment can be constipation or diarrhea. But the longer term of not fermenting and creating these short-chain fatty acids and having a healthy good bacteria population that's fed and growing is increased infection, toxins buildup, and the buildup of hormones. If your toxins and hormones can't break down, you feel sick, in pain, and have severe hormonal symptoms like weight gain. The last step always suffers the most because any step is broken before it impacts it. Most people have problems with the balance of good and bad bacteria in the gut. Most people have an infection in their gut. Most people have both these problems because they didn't address their digestion first.

There are additional lessons dedicated to infection and the microbiome.

**Everybody poops.** The consistency of stool is a fantastic health indicator that can offer valuable insights into your digestive and overall health. It serves as a direct reflection of how the gastrointestinal system is functioning and can reveal potential issues or imbalances. A healthy stool is typically soft, formed, and easy to pass, indicating that the digestive process has effectively absorbed nutrients and water while eliminating waste. Any significant deviation from this norm, whether in the form of loose, watery stools or hard, difficult-to-pass stools, is a sign that something is wrong with any of the number of steps in digestion. It can also be a powerful indicator of infection and even cancer.

Moreover, stool consistency can be an essential diagnostic tool for healthcare professionals. Persistent changes in stool consistency, such as chronic diarrhea or constipation, may indicate digestive disorders like irritable bowel syndrome (IBS), Crohn's disease, or celiac disease. Conversely, extremely pale or greasy stool might suggest issues with the liver or pancreas.

Monitoring stool consistency can empower individuals to proactively address their gastrointestinal health and seek medical attention when needed, helping prevent or manage potential health complications. Here's the Bristol scale chart that I love to share with my clients. There are images and descriptions to help you assess "the situation." In each section above, when you address digestion, for example, by taking a multi-phasic digestive product, some symptoms can have immediate change while others may be more long-term. Stool consistency is one of the indicators that, within 72 hours, things will change.

You can see it, and you can feel it. For example, if you are adequately hydrated, you will move from Type 1 further down the chart. If someone has poor fat digestion due to poor pancreas or liver function, they can move from Type 6-7 down within a few days. People may also notice increased regularity and even volume changes. I've often heard a client tell me within the first few days, "I have way more poop!" The point is, what you don't measure, you can't manage. Use your stool consistency as something you can measure to indicate change. Get encouraged and excited as you see this and other changes happening throughout your body!

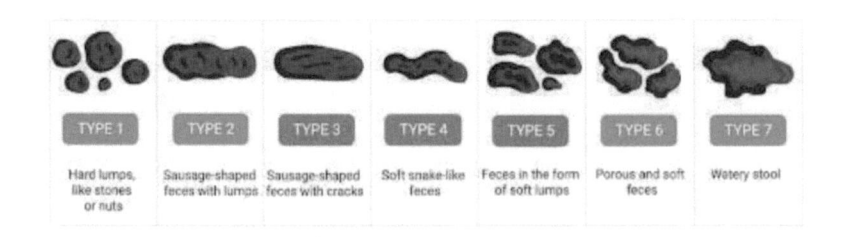

| TYPE 1 | TYPE 2 | TYPE 3 | TYPE 4 | TYPE 5 | TYPE 6 | TYPE 7 |
|--------|--------|--------|--------|--------|--------|--------|
| Hard lumps, like stones or nuts | Sausage-shaped feces with lumps | Sausage-shaped feces with cracks | Soft snake-like feces | Feces in the form of soft lumps | Porous and soft feces | Watery stool |

## Highlighting Downstream Effects From One Broken Step in Digestion, Low Stomach Acid

It's time to shine a spotlight again on low stomach acid, a seemingly minor issue with significant implications. Interestingly, I've found that 90% of individuals with chronic symptoms or diseases - including autoimmune conditions - struggle with low stomach acid. This striking fact suggests that low stomach acid may be the underpinning cause of many chronic illnesses.

The role of low stomach acid in our health is multifaceted, affecting more than just our gut. Surprisingly, it casts a shadow on conditions such as allergies, neuropathy, and even osteoporosis. Osteoporosis, characterized by brittle bones vulnerable to fractures, is commonly linked to hormonal fluctuations or insufficient calcium intake.

Yet, an often overlooked connection exists between this bone condition and reduced absorption of calcium and magnesium due to low stomach acid. In fact, low stomach acid is a plausible foundational cause of conditions like osteopenia and osteoporosis.

Acid plays an indispensable role in absorbing a spectrum of vitamins and minerals. Consider calcium and magnesium: without encountering the right level of stomach acid, their absorption is compromised. Drawing from chemistry, we know that pH levels influence the solubility of calcium. As such, the presence (or absence) of stomach acid directly alters the stomach's pH. Although many individuals consume calcium or magnesium supplements, their benefits might be negated without concurrent intake of a product that stimulates stomach acid production, such as DIGEST-IT. In this light, ensuring optimal stomach acid levels becomes crucial for overall bone health and nutrient absorption.

Consequently, those with low stomach acid may experience a variety of other symptoms due to impaired nutrient absorption. For example, they may find difficulty in digesting meat, not because of an allergic reaction or other common reasons, but due to this underlying acid deficiency.

If you don't have enough stomach acid, you don't digest meat well. It will sit in your stomach like a rock. Thomas had problems digesting meat. That was a telltale sign of low stomach acid.

Understanding the role of stomach acid in nutrient absorption can empower patients to tackle the root cause of their health issues. We can combat deficiencies, manage chronic diseases better, and improve overall well-being through education and awareness. It's time we give due attention to this 'minor' issue with significant implications for our health and revisit our understanding of chronic diseases in light of the crucial role played by stomach acid.

How many kids and adults have depression, anxiety, ADD, ADHD symptoms, or insomnia? Let's highlight another vitamin that doesn't get absorbed when stomach acid is low. Low B12 levels stemming from low stomach acid contribute to insomnia by lowering melatonin levels.

Melatonin can't be made without proper levels of B12. By ignoring the possibility of low stomach acid in children, we're disregarding an easily correctable cause of insomnia, anxiety, and ADD.

Nerves in the brain require B12 to heal and function properly. One of the underlying known causes of neuropathy, pain, or numbness is B12 deficiency. Yet, we have kids and adults with neurological symptoms, poor focus, ticks, and autism spectrum, and nobody is evaluating them for digestive problems that result in B12 deficiency and these symptoms. The standard of care says, just medicate these kids. Why not fix their stomach acid issues by giving them DIGEST-IT?

B12 deficiency from low stomach acid doesn't just cause mental health and brain-related focus problems; how about nerves causing chronic pain? Neuropathy causes pain in many ways, including conditions like sciatic pinched nerves like low back pain, carpal tunnel syndrome, TMJ in the jaw, and even facial pain, such as trigeminal neuralgia. Often, these pain syndromes remain mysterious to many doctors, with their root causes shrouded in uncertainty. But here's a surprising revelation: low stomach acid can be a hidden trigger for neuropathy. Nerves need B12 to absorb for proper nerve function and healing. Yet the most commonly prescribed treatment of nerve-induced pain doesn't address low stomach acid or vitamin B12 deficiency from its poor absorption.

On top of this, some of the medications we prescribe for chronic medical conditions deplete B12. We wonder why people with diabetes have nerve numbness and pain or neuropathy when the most frequently prescribed drug, Metformin, depletes B12. Proton-pump inhibitors (PPIs) like Prilosec and Nexium, which shut off stomach acid production, are known to impact B12 levels drastically. We wonder why people on these medications have high rates of gut infection, chronic pain, and insomnia.

## Learning Through My Own Experiences Road-Tested These Connections

In my personal health journey, I've deeply explored the intricacies of digestion. My experiences encompass neuropathy, TMJ jaw pain, facial discomfort, headaches, and persistent pain in my hands and forearms. Despite consulting numerous specialists, only a handful helped me consider unconventional causes for my pain. Surprisingly, none ever broached the topics of digestion or B12 deficiency.

Furthermore, none of these experts connected my issues to my history of autoimmunity. Research indicates that many individuals with autoimmune diseases suffer from low stomach acid. It's perplexing, then, why so many with autoimmune conditions grapple with chronic pain and consistently low B12 levels. It's essential to highlight that this isn't some unique, rare issue I'm facing alone. In fact, it's the predominant reason for chronic pain and neuropathy I observe among the clients we assist daily.

In my own experience with food allergies, not until I understood the role of these various steps in digestion and started taking supplementation did I see resolution of my eczema, hives, and chronic constipation from my food allergies. If I had to do it all over again, I'd tackle the digestion first in everybody to save them a lot of confusion, delay, and heartache along the way.

We have a specific process, Food Mapping, which I created to test a client's blood to figure out exactly which foods they are allergic to. This is beyond the allergist tests for IgE or anaphylactic-type allergies you already know—more on this in the lesson **Certainty About Food.** While many pin their hopes, thinking everything is related to these results, the truth is most people, by learning and tackling digestion first, have a massive reduction in their symptoms from digestive woes way before they even move on to food allergies.

While working with clients, I frequently stress the importance of distinguishing between allergic reactions to food and reactions stemming from digestive issues. Hence, the placement of this lesson early in the book. How many believe they're allergic to dairy? I once thought I was. Consuming dairy left me bloated and gassy. However, there's an intriguing point: if dairy causes these symptoms, but comprehensive Food Mapping tests indicate no allergy, it's likely due to lactose intolerance. This condition is a genetic absence of the enzyme needed to digest lactose, the sugar found in cow dairy products.

Thus, this response to dairy arises from a digestive incapability, not an allergy. In such cases, consuming a digestive enzyme with lactase can enable one to enjoy dairy without discomfort. Recognizing the difference between digestive issues and genuine allergies can be a game-changer.

Through my own pitfalls and challenging my own assumptions with science and actions, I was able to help myself, and others separate between digestive issues and allergic issues in response to eating.

# How to Start with the Right Digestive Support?

Let's go back to the symptoms we circled in Thomas's history.

- Knee and hip pain
- Weight gain
- Depression
- Indigestion
- Fullness after eating
- Bloating
- Eczema
- Dandruff

I've reviewed how low stomach acid can contribute to his knee and hip pain, indigestion, and bloating. I've shown how when someone has poor pancreas digestion, it can take the food a long time to get past the stomach to the small intestine; this was the cause of his fullness. Poor fat digestion from fatty liver from blood sugar swings (in the Blood Sugar Mastery lesson) and lack of digestive enzymes from his pancreas contributed to poor fat digestion and absorption. This low-fat absorption caused eczema, dandruff, and depression. Remember, your brain needs fat. His poor digestion led to poor nutrients in his large intestine, causing a decrease in the good bacteria and an increase in the harmful bacteria, causing poor fermentation.

When there's poor fermentation, hormones don't break down; they can build up, causing weight gain. (Estrogen dominance in men discussed in the Hormone lesson) Everything pointed to Thomas's digestion. Did you make some of those connections as you read through the different steps in digestion? Is this ringing a bell and feeling true about some of your own symptoms and their connection to digestion?

We've highlighted each step of digestion and action steps for each step. However, some of the steps require supplementation. When you are missing stomach acid, you need to take it. It's often genetically determined that people in a family all have low stomach acid or poor fat digestion.

Surgical intervention, the removal of digestive organs or parts of them, will require supplementation for life. For example, If your gallbladder was surgically removed, you can't secrete bile salts into the intestine to digest fats. You must take Ox Bile for life when you eat fat or else suffer from poor fat absorption into your body; the fat is needed for many functions and blood sugar stabilization. Some people with cancer or autoimmune diseases like Crohn's or ulcerative colitis have parts of their intestines removed. Would they be prone to have less length of their intestine for digestion and absorption? Would they need digestive support and probiotics to help increase the number of good bacteria in their gut? You betcha, and for life.

What's the critical takeaway from all this? Because of the high prevalence of multiple steps in digestion that can be genetically underperforming, a game changer would be to take a comprehensive multi-phasic digestive product like DIGEST-IT. Let's dive into why DIGEST-IT stands apart from many other digestive products. I've kissed a lot of frogs with recommendations for digestive products.

Firstly, it's easy to fall into the trap of thinking that you only need digestive enzymes or stomach acid. However, as you've just learned, digestion is a multifaceted process that often needs support at each stage— secondly, the ingredients matter. People with digestive issues often have allergies or sensitivities to certain supplements, medications, or foods. A supplement loaded with numerous ingredients could trigger these sensitivities. Unfortunately, many multi-phase digestive enzymes on the market pack an overwhelmingly long list of ingredients, creating intolerance issues for many individuals I've recommended. This led me to create a product with minimal yet highly effective ingredients that cover every step.

Enter DIGEST-IT. Most people can easily tolerate it, and its efficacy is impressive. There are too many testimonials to count on how life-changing this product has been. The take-home message here? Start with DIGEST-IT. With small meals, take one; with larger meals, take two. Pay attention to your body's responses – these invaluable data points often provide more insight than standard medical tests.

Remember, the key is understanding the various symptoms at each step and adjusting the dosage as needed.

When you browse our website, www.mymdshop.com, you'll find a broad spectrum of digestive products tailored to various needs, allergies, tolerability issues, and age groups. We offer chewable tablets, a godsend for children and adults who struggle with swallowing capsules. Just the other day, a mom told us her four-year-old reminds her to give her the "food vitamins." The four-year-old can tell a big difference when she takes it and, as a result, will ask for it. It goes to show that doing something that works is the best way to get someone else to keep doing something.

In our programs, depending on people's reaction to taking DIGEST-IT, the response or lack thereof provides further data from your body that helps us troubleshoot how to play with digestive supports. In our GI essentials, there are multiple other products that can be added for digestive support. The part of teaching I enjoy most and has been the most fun for me is that, as a physician, we're able to take the additional data of someone's response or lack of a response to a supplement and teach people how to use that information to increase, decrease or switch supplementation.

Here are some additional products often used to troubleshoot or to be added based on symptoms and history:

**Ox Bile:** for someone without a gallbladder or who finds that fatty meals are poorly tolerated, they may add ox bile in addition to DIGEST-IT to help digest higher-fat meals.

- It is derived from a bovine source and freeze-dried (lyophilized) to maintain its biological activity. Ox Bile is a suitable supplement to the liver's production of bile.
- Recommendation: take 1 or 2 capsules with DIGEST-IT to aid in the digestion of high-fat meals.

**Quercetin-Bromelain Forte:** for those with known mast cell or histamine intolerance or who can't tolerate supplements with a large number of ingredients. This product is designed for those people to take if they can't tolerate DIGEST-IT. The high amount of both quercetin and bromelain can digest and lower histamine levels.

- Quercetin-Bromelain Forté provides a mixture of proteolytic enzymes and bioflavonoids that help regulate the immune cytokine response.
- Quercetin is a powerful bioflavonoid that protects cells and tissues against free radicals.
- Bromelain, papain, and pancreatin provide a mixture of protein-specific and other enzymes that help ensure the proper breakdown of protein molecules that may otherwise cause irritation.† Vitamin C, buffered with magnesium to eliminate acidity, supports histamine metabolism, detoxification processes, and collagen synthesis.

**Histaway:** for those who after eating a known allergen or who still experience histamine-related symptoms after eating, use of this product after eating (does not replace DIGEST-IT) utilizes a different mechanism to lower histamine levels after the food has been ingested, and the histamine response is already underway. Many clients with mast cell or histamine intolerance have found this product to be life-saving.

- HISTAWAY is a patented enzyme formula containing diamine oxidase (DAO)—the main enzyme responsible for the degradation of ingested histamine.
- This enzyme has been clinically tested and found to break down food- derived histamine in the digestive tract. DAO is not absorbed and does not have systemic activity.
- Histaway does not manage or address antibody-related or IgE-related food allergies. Take one to two capsules no more than 15 minutes before the consumption of histamine-rich foods or after. It may take up to 10 capsules a day to manage histamine-related symptoms as a result of food consumption.

## Action Steps

1. Dilution is digestion; drink as you eat your food.
2. Chew each bite ten times. Mechanical digestion of breaking down food into smaller and smaller digestible particles is key.
3. Take a multi-phasic digestive product like DIGEST-IT, one for small and two for larger meals, as a starting point.
4. Supplements mentioned are available at www.mymdshop.com

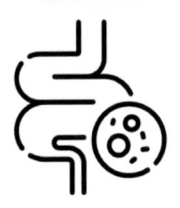

# LESSON 3:
# THE GUT: GETTING OFF THE MERRY-GO-ROUND

*"Change the inner landscape, and you'll find the external transformed."*

-Maggie Yu MD IFMCP

The gut microbiome plays a pivotal role in overall health, influencing everything from digestion to immunity. We'll be exploring this "earth" inside you and how it can get into dysfunction when the inhabitants are not in balance with each other. With an imbalanced environment and other ongoing assaults, invaders can easily take hold. We'll be exploring the effect this has and how it has led infection to become such a rampant yet hidden epidemic.

## The Gut Microbiome: Our Internal Ecosystem

Imagine, if you will, your gut as a microcosm of Earth itself. The term "microbiome" might sound enigmatic, but let's simply look at it as a system of inhabitants living inside you. It consists of various bacterial species, each with its unique role. Keystone species, in particular, are crucial for the gut's overall health, aiding in functions like digestion and blood sugar balance. Let's explore this rich internal ecosystem, your mini Earth.

In this microscopic Earth within you, just like on our planet, a diverse array of bacterial species calls it home. Much like Earth's ecosystems, your gut has its own balance to maintain. It's a bustling place where conflicts arise, and invaders seek to disrupt the harmony, akin to migratory forces altering geographical landscapes.

Now, picture the gut microbiome as a bustling city with various key players, the keystone species. These are the unsung heroes, the utility workers, teachers, and police officers of this tiny world. They perform vital roles, from fortifying the protective mucus layer to aiding in digestion and regulating blood sugar levels. Ensuring their presence in both abundance and diversity is essential, for it is this diversity that underpins your overall well-being. You want a high number of utility workers in all trades, all functions working hard at their own jobs and to better the environment for all the other inhabitants. Keystone species are essential for this reason. You not only want a high number of them, but you want a high diversity, all different types of them. In fact, you want as many different types of utility workers as possible so that every function imaginable has a key player on the job.

## The Gut-Brain Connection

Stress doesn't just weigh on the mind; it also reshapes the landscape of our gut. Persistent emotional turmoil, such as chronic anxiety or worry, can notably influence the balance of our gut bacteria. This can result in a decline in bacterial diversity, allowing certain bacteria to flourish while others wane.

At the heart of this is how stress affects our nervous system. You see, stress kicks our "fight or flight" response into gear, governed by the sympathetic nervous system. On the other side of the coin is the parasympathetic system, the "calm and rest" response that promotes digestion. With chronic stress dampening this restful state, both digestion and nutrient absorption suffer.

Moreover, stress unleashes a surge of hormones like adrenaline and cortisol. Over time, these hormones amplify inflammation in the gut, which may exacerbate conditions like irritable bowel syndrome (IBS) and inflammatory bowel disease (IBD). It's no surprise, then, that many individuals with IBS and IBD also report elevated levels of anxiety and stress. In essence, stress can amplify the severity of these conditions.

But the story doesn't end there. Enter the Gut-Brain Connection. This symbiotic relationship ensures the gut and brain communicate seamlessly. However, stress can muddle this dialogue, leading to altered gut motility, digestion anomalies, and even the emergence of food allergies. It's compelling to observe that individuals diagnosed with food allergies, IBS, or IBD often report chronic stress, which further underscores the imbalance of bacteria in their gut.

As we navigate this connection between the gut and our emotions, the message is clear: Our mental well-being is inextricably linked to the health of our gut. Curious? Let's continue to explore this further.

## Gut Dysbiosis, Disruptors

But there's another side to this microbial tale—the disruptors. These are the species that, when they are in check and in small numbers, are just fine. It's like a concert with a mixed group, and the police have reasonable crowd control. But when in excessive numbers, some of the revelers, these disruptors, can upset the balance of power and the direction of the crowd's behavior. They're called imbalanced bacteria that can be present in small numbers. They might not hold keystone roles, but their sheer abundance can throw the entire system into chaos, affecting both the numbers and the functional diversity of the keystone species. The delicate equilibrium of your gut "Earth" is at stake.

Under these imbalanced species, in stool testing, I have found that there are a lot of bacteria from the mouth, gums, dental flora, sinuses, and ears that seed into the gut. These imbalanced bacteria can enter through ingestion, but they are also constantly being seeded from problems with dental, sinus, and ear health, creating ongoing imbalances. Sometimes, it's just a matter of the right person in the wrong place. Some bacteria are just fine sitting in your dental microbiome, but if there are digestive problems or an extremely high number of them entering the intestines where they don't belong, they will influence the delicate balance in the gut microbiome and disrupt the behavior and function of the other species that are working there.

# What are Gut Infections

Lastly, let's talk about infectious species, the invaders—a group that certainly doesn't belong at the gut's grand banquet or, when present in excessive numbers, creates a war zone. These infectious species can be bacteria, viruses, parasites, or fungi that overwhelm the gut's cellular defenses, causing what we commonly recognize as infections. In an active infection, the invaders are killing the inhabitants of a city. They replace the keystone species with more of their own. This invasion or infection stops vital functions and decreases the population, just like what happens in a war.

The key workers in utilities, water, gas, electric, and waste management are attacked, and many of them are killed. Replaced by thugs whose only interest is to populate themselves and not perform any duties or provide any services for the city. Piece by piece, organ by organ, step by step through the length of the intestines, these infectious invaders march through, and not only do they attack and kill inhabitants, but the structures along their march are destroyed. Key structures like the water tower are dismantled. These structures are your cell lining in the intestinal. Imagine that your gut cells are like a high defense wall against invaders.

## Understanding Leaky Gut

Once the good bacteria, the utility workers, are killed, the invader advances towards the wall and starts to attack your own intestinal mucosa cells that line your intestine. These cells act as the wall, and they are linked to each other arm-in-arm in bonds called healthy tight junctions, as you see on the left of the diagram.

**LEAKY GUT SYNDROME**

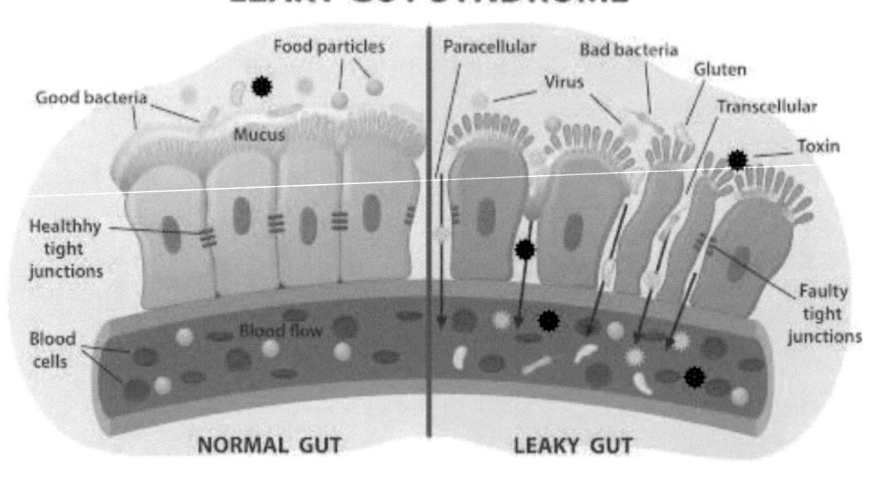

*Normal Gut | Leaky Gut*

Labels: Good bacteria, Mucus, Healthy tight junctions, Blood cells, Blood flow, Food particles, Paracellular, Bad bacteria, Virus, Gluten, Transcellular, Toxin, Faulty tight junctions

Imagine your gut as a fortress designed to keep harmful invaders at bay. But when an infection strikes, it's as though the fortress walls are breached, allowing unwelcome elements to seep through.

When these invaders penetrate the protective layer of good bacteria and mucus lining, they damage the gut lining cells and break their tight junctions. This compromised barrier acts like a castle wall with gaping holes, permitting these malicious agents unrestricted access into the bloodstream and, from there, to the rest of the body.

This breach is why individuals with gut infections often exhibit heightened allergic reactions. Their systems become inundated with foreign entities, leading their immune systems to produce histamines in defense. These histamines, the body's reaction to unfamiliar intruders, signify its relentless effort to maintain balance.

Substances from the gut then cascade into the bloodstream, radiating throughout the body and initiating a domino effect of health repercussions. It's evident, recalling our previous discussion on digestion, that those with this condition, commonly known as leaky gut syndrome, face challenges in digesting and absorbing nutrients. By recognizing the profound role of the gut microbiome and its vulnerability to infections, we can better appreciate the intricacies of this health narrative.

Take, for instance, the notorious trio of H.pylori, SIBO, or Candida. When any of these invade your gut, they arrive in such formidable numbers that they can infect, dismantle, and overpopulate to squeeze keystone species out of the picture and destroy the environment, triggering many other symptoms or diseases like irritable bowel syndrome, fibromyalgia, mast cell, and histamine intolerance. One of the underlying mechanisms for why one person would always be in a pain flare or an autoimmune disease flare is the continued infection and destruction happening in their gut, triggering many other deleterious results throughout the body.

COVID-19 has proven to be more than just a respiratory adversary; it significantly impacts the digestive system as well. A myriad of patients with COVID-19 have reported gastrointestinal symptoms such as nausea, stomach discomfort, diarrhea, and constipation. In my work with post-COVID clients, stool tests frequently indicate considerable disturbances in their gut bacteria. Many of the prolonged symptoms these individuals face, often termed "long-haul" symptoms, align closely with the manifestations of a leaky gut. Affected individuals commonly report chronic fatigue, irritable bowel syndrome, heightened allergic responses, and difficulties in maintaining stable blood pressure. Consequently, they experience dizziness, nausea, vertigo, and irregularities in both blood pressure and heart rate.

Viruses, such as COVID-19, adenovirus, and norovirus, can directly assault your gut's cells, hijacking them into viral replication factories. This viral insurgency leads to a surge in virus production, further exacerbating the gut's turmoil. It's a vivid example of how a viral infection can have a profound impact on both gut bacteria and the gut's cellular harmony.

In summary, Infections, as war invaders, tend to leave quite a mess behind with leaky gut. They trigger cell death, unleashing a cascade of toxins that wreak havoc and disrupt the gut's delicate ecosystem. This affects not only the keystone species but also their critical operations within the gut.

As a result of the loss of the inhabitants, the structural integrity of your gut lining cells becomes compromised, creating a condition of leaky gut. A leaky gut is an open door for invaders to go past your immune defense straight into your bloodstream. It becomes a microbial cascade with enormous consequences on many symptoms, including pain, immune system, allergies, brain function, mood, and cardiovascular system. The understanding of this concept is the key to this lesson.

## Infection is the Modern Plague. Why?

*Illene, a decade-long scleroderma, an autoimmune disease affecting connective tissue on skin, lungs, gut, and joints, had trouble swallowing, chronic pain throughout her body, and nerve pain in her arms and legs. She complained of being constipated, having only one to two bowel movements a week. She had tight skin, breathlessness with shortness of breath, recurring rashes, and itching that kept her up at night. She had seen multiple rheumatologists and was on several medications for her scleroderma.*

*One of her medications is a steroid called prednisone. This anti-inflammatory medication, with many side effects, is something that she has been working on weaning down. Yet her lung capacity was at about 50%, and she needed to be on oxygen. Despite being on the medications, her symptoms over the past several years only got worse. Worse yet, several times a year, she would contract an upper respiratory infection and would end up taking antibiotics about twice a year.*

*When I met her, no one had tested her hormones; she was perimenopausal. She had severe brain fog and insomnia. She also had a long history of heavy and irregular periods and fibroids. She was not a diabetic, so no one discussed or explored the blood sugar fluctuations that she was experiencing. She also had no idea what foods were triggering her swallowing and skin tightness.*

*While going through the program, she saw her pain decrease, the rashes began to be less frequent, and about six months later, the nerve zaps in her arms and legs began to subside. But something still wasn't right. Her lung capacity was sitting at about 60%, and she still needed to be on oxygen.*

*It was discovered while working with us that she had an underlying fungal infection, Candida. Fungal organisms are known to trigger increased allergic reactions and pain. After clearing her infection with her, she now reports that her lung capacity has hit 90% several years later.*

Illene's journey, familiar to many, beautifully encapsulates the various lessons we've traversed in preceding chapters. With each page turned, you may have discerned how every lesson played a pivotal role in carving her path to wellness. Yet, it's vital to underscore the pronounced influence of infections on a spectrum of chronic health symptoms. Let's spotlight certain aspects of her history and symptoms to gauge why an infection might be the lingering obstacle in her pursuit of optimal health. Curious about the intricacies? Let's unravel them together.

Highlight the following history and symptoms in Illene's case study:

- History of autoimmune disease, scleroderma
- Chronic pain throughout her body
- Neuropathy, nerve pain in arms and legs
- Frequent Upper Respiratory Infections
- Trouble swallowing
- Constipation
- Itching

- Taking several immune-suppressing medications, including prednisone
- Hormone imbalance symptoms like brain fog and insomnia

You might believe that the invention of antibiotics marked the conclusion of our fight against infections. Dive deeper. Not only are we entangled in this ongoing battle, but in some areas, we're falling behind. Every day, clinics and hospitals distribute antibiotics, sometimes even preemptively. The reality is undeniable: antibiotics are overused. This over-reliance disrupts the balance between good and bad bacteria in our systems. Antibiotics, unfortunately, don't discriminate. While they might eliminate the bacteria causing an ailment, they also diminish your body's beneficial bacteria.

While doctor-prescribed antibiotics come with their risks, they're not the only threat to our bacterial balance. Our food plays a significant role. Livestock like cows, chickens, pigs, and fish are frequently reared in densely populated enclosures, leading to an uptick in disease. To manage this, industries heavily medicate these animals with antibiotics, creating antibiotic resistance. These antibiotics then enter our systems when we consume the meat. The resulting antibiotic resistance paves the way for powerful multi-resistant organisms that defy our medical knowledge.

Moreover, our challenges aren't just limited to well-known infections. Sneaky bacteria like H.pylori often go undetected, mimicking milder conditions such as heartburn. Many, like Illene, have their gut flora disrupted by antibiotics, making them vulnerable to these resistant organisms.

Often, mainstream medicine misinterprets certain conditions, leading to mismanagement and exacerbating issues. An example is the misconception that heartburn stems from high stomach acid levels, prompting prescriptions for acid-reducing medications. This not only paves the way for harmful organisms but also overlooks the root causes of the ailment.

Moreover, infections are increasingly prevalent in our narrative of chronic health. From Candida and Lyme to Epstein-Barr virus and long haul COVID, these infections are alarmingly recurrent. They often lead to severe conditions like autoimmune diseases, fibromyalgia, and chronic fatigue.

## Getting to the Root

But the burning question remains: are infections the primary culprits or mere repercussions of pre-existing body imbalances? My client's experiences suggest the latter. Infections often result from ignored issues, whether they be digestive complications, food intolerances, or hormonal discrepancies. Those with autoimmune diseases, for instance, have compromised immune systems, making them more susceptible to infections.

Tackling infections without understanding their origins is a fruitless endeavor. A well-rounded, integrated approach requires us to shift our focus from the symptoms to the root causes. By altering the environment that breeds these infections, we can prevent their recurrence.

Consider Illene's story as a poignant lesson. Prednisone suppressed her immune system, making her susceptible to infections. The antibiotics she took further skewed her internal balance. Only by addressing these underlying problems could Illene restore her health and eradicate her infections. It's crucial to determine and address the root causes first. This story underscores a fundamental principle: sequencing matters.

It's not just about treating infections; it's about doing it right. What are the pivotal steps both Illene and you should prioritize?

**Digestion:** Every step in the digestive process is vital in producing substances that both break down food and defend against infections. For instance, stomach acid, much like vinegar's disinfectant qualities, acts as a barrier against infections. Prioritizing and supporting every stage of digestion is paramount. Please go back to the digestion lesson. Ilene had severe bloating and difficulty swallowing; she learned this was due to low stomach acid.

**Food Allergens:** Imagine the potential ripple effect in your gut when faced with undetected food allergens. This hidden battlefield creates a unique opportunity for infections to thrive. With certainty, utilizing an accurate system to test for and understand food sensitivities, like the Food Mapping System I created, can lead to impressive strides to turn it around. Unknown to many and often overlooked by physicians, undetected food allergies lead to unintentionally consuming problematic foods. This places our intestines in a perpetual state of unrest. It's a war zone fighting allergens all the time!

Such an agitated and compromised environment lights a torch for opportunistic infections to take hold gleefully. I always say when there's a war zone, the thugs love to come in. They loot and thrive, and they increase in numbers. That's your gut full of allergens. Without a deep understanding of food allergens, this environment remains unchanged, perpetuating the gut's role as an inviting haven for microorganisms. They love to come back over and over again to an environment that is inviting them. This environment must be changed to change its inhabitants. Illene was sensitive to gluten and corn. Eliminating both caused her swallowing and shortness of breath to improve after just a few months. The itchy rashes are now entirely gone because she's no longer consuming allergens.

**Blood Sugar Stabilization:** This is a reminder of why blood sugar mastery is required for any chronic health symptom. As it relates to infection, elevated blood sugar levels provide a feast for infectious organisms, from Lyme to E. Coli, allowing them to thrive. We already know how much COVID-19 loves those who have diabetes. But you don't have to be a diabetic to have high sugar surges that feed any infections. As discussed in the blood sugar lesson, the plummet of that high sugar to low causes a devastating blow to hormone production, hormone breakdown, liver function, and toxin breakdown. In any infection, the sugars will increase the numbers of those organisms rapidly, and when the blood sugar plunges, many of those organisms can also die.

During these daily swings in infection, when organisms die, they frequently trigger a condition called "die-off." When thousands die, they split open, releasing lipopolysaccharides (LPS). LPS flows in the bloodstream and throughout the body, causing the liver to get inflamed, as does the rest of your body. Infection flares up and down is the trigger for many of the physical symptoms and other problems going on. The bottom line is blood sugar swings fuel infection and its various downstream symptoms. These blood sugar swings will cause tremendous swings in the number and activity of the infectious organisms. So, blood sugar mastery must come first. One of the challenges of dealing with infection without blood sugar mastery is the tremendous amount of die-off symptoms that complicate treatment and the ability to stay on treatment.

This case study highlights the best approach to infection is to address other lessons involving digestion, blood sugar, and food allergens first. Order truly matters. Doing the right thing at the wrong time is still the wrong thing.

The steps above are key to making the next steps in this lesson the right thing at the right time to set up for the eradication of infection and the invaders effectively. Let's expand on what's the proper order to deal with infection.

## Order Matters

Imagine the overwhelming feeling of confronting countless providers, antibiotics, supplements, and thousands of Google research to find ways to address a stubborn recurring infection that nobody believes you have. That's the typical journey of most people I meet who understand they have a gut infection but don't know the best way to tackle it. Meanwhile, their overall health symptoms are staying the same or getting worse. The biggest frustration is the lack of clarity and the repeating cycle of this. Even when someone thinks I've gotten rid of an infection, it keeps coming back!

The fundamental lesson about infection? Begin by altering the environment within. Reframe your internal ecosystem, emphasizing its structural integrity, utility, quality, and inherent collaboration. In cultivating such terrain, you bolster your defenses, minimizing disruptions and intrusions from both external invaders and any antibiotics you might ingest. However, when discord does arise, many merely target the intruders, neglecting the need to restore their internal landscape to its initial robust state. This oversight paves the way for perpetual battles as these unwelcome guests return in relentless waves.

Too often, individuals approach us having felt unheard by their mainstream healthcare providers for years. Many traditional medical professionals, be they family physicians, internal medicine specialists, or gastroenterologists, remain skeptical about the existence of gut infections. They're similarly dismissive of the "leaky gut" concept despite mounting evidence confirming its legitimacy. Their toolkit seems limited: when confronted with an infection, their default response is often to prescribe more antibiotics. Such treatments, as we've discussed, unsettle the gut's equilibrium, eliminating both harmful and beneficial bacteria. This limited perspective, akin to viewing every problem as a nail simply because one possesses a hammer, is constraining. Yet, driven by genuine curiosity, functional medicine practitioners consistently diagnose and address infections.

Many seek the expertise of functional medicine professionals undergoing advanced diagnostic tests that not only identify specific pathogens but also shed light on digestive processes, gut hormones, and the overall health of one's gut lining. After receiving their diagnosis, patients often invest significant resources into treatments, from specialty diets and IV therapies to medications and supplements. While these treatments can be incredibly effective, a recurring challenge is the persistence of these infections. Have you, dear reader, sought treatment for conditions like Candida, Lyme, or SIBO multiple times? You're certainly not alone. We interact with countless individuals sharing your experiences, daily.

The missing piece of this intricate puzzle? An emphasis on reshaping the internal environment either before or concurrently with infection treatment to thwart recurring episodes.

For effective and lasting infection management, the preliminary steps must encompass:

- Digestion Enhancement
- Food Mapping for allergen identification and elimination
- Mastery of Blood Sugar Regulation
- Strengthening the Gut Microbiome

These guidelines sketch out a sequence to prioritize. When one commits to this strategic order, they'll likely observe a natural reduction in both gut-related complications and infection occurrences.

*"Don't put the cart before the horse. Order Matters"*
-**Maggie Yu MD IFMCP**

# Fermentation: The Unsung Hero of Gut Health

Fermentation is the silent champion of your gut, a vital process that often goes unnoticed. Yet, it plays a central role in everything from hormone balance to toxin breakdown and even digestion itself. Think of it as the grand finale in the digestive orchestra, the last act before the curtain falls. This was discussed as one of the final steps in the digestion lesson. We are going into more depth here.

So, what exactly is fermentation? It's a remarkable process where proteins, fats, and carbohydrates are transformed into simpler molecules, all thanks to the orchestration of bacteria, yeast, and other microorganisms in your gut. This transformation yields products that are nothing short of magical—they help heal leaky gut, provide a source of energy, assist in breaking down hormones and toxins, and nourish the growth of beneficial microorganisms.

Enter prebiotics, a form of fiber that serves as fuel for these microorganism marvels, accelerating fermentation. Among the treasures produced by fermentation are short-chain fatty acids (SCFAs), which not only fuel the microorganisms but also serve as sustenance for your own body's cells. These SCFAs are instrumental in breaking down hormones and toxins.

Among them, the versatile butyrate stands as a key player, crucial for gut healing, combating brain fog, and tackling chronic fatigue.

But the wonders don't stop there. SCFAs also venture into the world of nerves, promoting their growth and healing. This revelation holds particular significance for those grappling with neuropathy, brain fog, ADHD, depression, or anxiety. As it turns out, glial cells in the brain and nerve cells throughout the body rely on fermentation products for their growth and repair.

And here's where things get even more fun. Large intestinal bacteria join the party as hormone breakdown experts. While your liver initiates hormone breakdown, gut bacteria in the intestines take it a step further through hormone detoxification, all part of the fermentation process. So, it's safe to say if you don't ferment well, you can't balance your hormones. This is discussed in the hormone lesson, as well.

Why is this crucial? Well, the efficient breakdown of hormones matters—a lot. Specific hormone-breakdown molecules can be downright toxic. The faster your body detoxifies and the more good bacteria there are to ferment in your large intestine, the more efficiently you'll break down hormones into their less active forms. This means you can bid farewell to them more effectively, resulting in improved hormone balance and reduced toxicity from excess estrogen or xenoestrogens.

Many of the hormonal symptoms you experience are a result of the toxic buildup from excess hormones not adequately broken down in the final step of fermentation. The same can be said for all the toxins that are broken down by fermentation. It's safe to say that you can't detox without fermentation. Illene had an abnormally high amount of estrogen in comparison to her progesterone. She was in a state of hormone excess, with one hormone overpowering another. Estrogen dominance will trigger symptoms of brain fog and insomnia, and this is a direct result of the problem with fermentation and hormone breakdown she was having.

But the impact of these intricate processes isn't confined to digestion, hormone balance, or detoxification alone. They reach into the brain and neurological functions, influencing brain activity. This can lead to symptoms like brain fog and ADD. Fermentation affects mood. I've also discussed how chronically feeling stress affects the gut bacteria balance in the gut-brain connection.

So, if the fermenters are out of balance and their job is out of balance, you can see how stress and mood affect the bacteria that ferment. The changes in the products they produce and remove, go right back to the brain to further cause changes to the brain. Irritated nerves throughout the body and in the brain affect our brain neurotransmitters and the hormones that the grain makes, shaping our daily thought processes, focus, and mood.

8 Out of the Box Ways to Transform Your Health
From Confusion to Confidence: The Playbook for Whole Body Wellness

And remember, the scope of fermentation's influence on health is huge. There isn't one lesson here that gut bacteria and fermentation doesn't affect. We've only scratched the surface. However, infectious invaders will kill the good bacteria and disrupt fermentation. Let's discuss the how and the action steps to improve fermentation and to build a better microbiome, the Earth inside you!

## How to Build Your Microbiome "Earth"

**Populate with probiotics.** Probiotics are good bacteria that contribute to a number of keystone species and the health of other keystone species. Probiotics matter, but the problem is people choose probiotics based on marketing and misinformation. Some best-selling probiotics on Amazon have misleading names because people think the number of good bacteria is what matters. You can have 100 billion colonies, but they're useless if they don't do anything in your intestines or contribute to the keystone species. They're cheap to make, and companies market them based on quantity rather than effectiveness.

This is why it's not true when someone says you can just eat yogurt for probiotics. Yogurt contains strains that are great at making yogurt. They are not necessarily the medically studied strains backed by data that do the job you need them to do specifically. They may be generally helpful. But often have little activity to promote the growth of keystone species. They're just strains that help yogurt companies produce yogurt. Yogurt companies use these strains to ferment the sugars in milk to create yogurt as a product.

Eating yogurt is helpful but can provide limited specific health benefits.

For those seriously committed to making health choices for longevity based on data and what creates the most impact, start thinking about the specific bacterial strains you need to take as a probiotic.

There are many functions keystone species bacteria need to do, such as balancing hormones, digesting food, performing fermentation, balancing blood sugar, aiding weight loss, and improving mood and focus. Some strains promote balance in the immune system, decrease histamines, and even promote an anti-cancer environment. More and more data is defining precisely what those strains are. Data-driven probiotic therapy or specific strain probiotic therapy to perform specific jobs is essential. The vast majority of probiotics being sold right now don't do many of the things you need, making them useless and expensive. Even if bought at a low price, it's a waste of money if they don't do the job they're supposed to.

Investing in probiotics can often raise eyebrows. Yet, consider the immense value they bring when tailored to individual needs. Imagine a probiotic specifically designed to combat histamines and food allergies. Such a formulation could drastically enhance your daily life by alleviating unpredictable ailments like diarrhea, which can be disruptive to work and travel. Certain bacterial strains even have the potential to lower histamine levels in foods, thus minimizing allergic responses, even when one consumes potential allergens. This underscores the importance of selecting probiotics with a clear objective in mind.

Probiotics can be an effective way to promote gut health and overall well-being. At MY.MD Bio-Therapeutic, we offer a range of probiotics designed to address specific health needs, such as balancing blood sugar and decreasing allergies.

Our recommended regimen includes rotating at least two specific probiotics, such as:

**PRO-FLORA AI+** provides support for both the upper and lower GI tract for digestive and immune health. This concentrated formula supplies a proprietary blend of the most beneficial probiotic strains to transform the health of your intestinal tract.

- Helps Maintain a Healthy Intestinal Microbiome
- Supports Bowel Regularity
- Supports Gastrointestinal-Based Immunity

It is ideal for individuals seeking a well-rounded supplement to support a healthy balance of intestinal flora, cellular health, and immune health.

**PRO-FLORA AI+** features four probiotic strains, including the extensively studied HN019 strain of Bifidobacterium lactis, plus Saccharomyces boulardii (Sb), a non-pathogenic yeast, to further complement healthy gastrointestinal ecology as a powerful species to combat infection in challenging times. Lactobacillus Plantarum is clinically shown to decrease histamines and combat insulin resistance.

And...

**PRO-FLORA GI** is an extensively researched strain of "friendly" bacteria, LP299V®, designed to help

- Relieve occasional irritation and bowel discomfort
- Support the integrity of the gastrointestinal barrier
- Support immune health.

Ideal for individuals with irritable bowel syndrome, leaky gut, and those struggling with gut infections.

An important concept is the introduction of variety and specific strains that do specific jobs. It's important to avoid using the same probiotic or bacteria all the time. To increase gut biodiversity, I recommend rotating multiple probiotics. But be selective about the exact strains you want to introduce into your regimen to help with improving the keystone species that do specific functions.

It's important to note that imbalanced or infectious bacteria in your gut can lead to various health issues, such as autoimmune diseases, thyroid conditions, and colon cancer. Therefore, taking quality probiotics targeted for protection to preserve those functions can play a crucial role in maintaining gut health and overall well-being.

We believe in taking well-studied and data-driven probiotics to help decrease symptoms, reduce chronic disease, and promote longevity. Additionally, our recommended soil-based probiotics can significantly improve gut diversity and have antimicrobial properties.

**Action step:** Rotate quality probiotics like PRO-FLORA AI+ and GI to increase gut diversity and keystone species. Visit our probiotic collection to select probiotics based on your goals.

**Nurture the beneficial bacteria in your gut.** Simply taking probiotics is not enough; these beneficial bacteria require the right environment and nutrients to thrive and work effectively. This means we need to feed probiotics with prebiotics – essentially, fibers and resistant starches. These aren't rapidly absorbed in your gut; they travel to your large intestine, nourishing your gut bacteria and promoting healthy fermentation. Hence, a high-fiber diet is vital.

Consuming at least six cups of fruits and vegetables a day, including hormone-balancing cruciferous vegetables, is highly beneficial. Incorporating fiber into your meals can be straightforward; for instance, batch-cooked tray bakes of root vegetables or cabbage slaws are delicious, fiber-rich options.

Medical foods can be a practical solution for those finding it challenging to boost fiber intake. FIBER PLUS, for example, provides specific fiber types that serve as prebiotics. Adding a daily scoop to your smoothie can significantly increase your gut bacteria's prebiotic supply.

**FIBER PLUS** is the ultimate fiber product. It is a comprehensive product that contains 12 different types of fiber and none of the allergenic proteins or harsh, irritating components commonly found in other fiber products on the market.

This product was designed with the features of the Paleolithic diet in mind, for which human physiology may be best adapted. FIBER PLUS could be a useful tool to help support proper weight management, glucose metabolism, and lipid metabolism.

Additionally, LOVE MY GREENS, a greens powder, supplies ample fiber and phytonutrients found in colorful fruits and vegetables. These phytonutrients offer a myriad of benefits, from cancer prevention and anti-inflammation to supporting cardiovascular and brain health.

**LOVE MY GREENS** is a greens powder densely packed with high oxygen radical absorbance capacity (ORAC) valued vegetables, cleansing alkalizing grass juices, and a proprietary blend of fruits and berries. Besides being phytonutrient-rich, the orange-cranberry flavor tastes terrific, thanks to the inclusion of inulin, a natural polysaccharide prebiotic fiber, along with a splash of stevia. This adds a subtly sweet flavor to Love My Greens, as inulin does not impact blood sugar levels the same way as many other sweeteners. Inulin is a soluble fiber that dissolves easily in water, making Love My Greens simple to mix into any beverage.

**Action Step:** Prioritizing fiber-rich food. Biohack your fiber intake by supplementing with medical foods like FIBER PLUS and LOVE MY GREENS into your smoothie, soups, or sauces.

**Eat fermented foods.** Fermented foods provide us with beneficial bacteria and the short-chain fatty acids (SCFAs) these gut microbes produce. These SCFAs play a crucial role in our body, from breaking down hormones and toxins to improving our overall gut health. With minimal downside, integrating more fermented foods into our diets is a simple way to boost our health. However, it's worth noting that those with severe allergies, mast cell activation, or histamine intolerance might need to moderate their intake due to the potential elevation of histamines in fermented foods.

For the vast majority, incorporating fermented foods is highly beneficial. Foods like sauerkraut, yogurt, and kimchi are nutrient-dense and straightforward to integrate into daily meals. Take kimchi, for example - a true nutritional powerhouse. This fermented cabbage dish delivers three benefits: it's rich in fiber, is a nutritious cruciferous vegetable, and carries all the advantages of fermentation.

Plus, it's easy to make at home! Incorporating fermented foods into your diet is a surefire way to enhance your health journey. There are many online recipes and videos on fermenting various foods, or you can purchase them.

Now, fermentation is different from pickling. Fermentation actually uses bacteria to ferment the cabbage, for example, in sauerkraut, and then it tastes sour. So it's fermented, not pickled. Pickling is different because it uses acid and heat to make and preserve something sour. There's a big difference between the two. There are companies now that make traditionally pickled foods, but they ferment them, such as fermented pickles or olives. It's fascinating that people are starting to understand that eating fermented foods has tons of health benefits. Kombucha is also a fermented food, so drinking kombucha is a great idea, but make sure it is low to none in added sugar.

Nourish your beneficial gut bacteria by delighting them with fermented foods. Many of these foods also boast high fiber content, elegantly addressing three key points in one go. First, they supply prebiotics; second, they deliver ample fiber; and third, they introduce a fascinating variety of fermentation-derived nutrients. By making fermented foods a mainstay of your diet, you effectively optimize your gut health and foster a vibrant internal ecosystem.

Make, buy, and eat more fermented foods like sauerkraut, kimchi, and kombucha.

**You've got to poop every day.** There are numerous ways to allow toxins to infiltrate our systems, and some are created in our bodies, including certain hormone-breakdown products that can cause hormonal imbalances. The cumulative effect of these toxins is profound, and inadequate bowel movements further complicate their management. For instance, infrequent bowel movements can increase your toxic load significantly. I've previously discussed this issue in social media training videos, comparing the toxic load of individuals who eliminate daily versus those who do so weekly. The latter group's toxic load is potentially many times higher, emphasizing the importance of daily bowel movements. Yes, at least once a day for the best toxin-clearing machine that you are.

Elimination is vital in toxin management - it's how we expel the toxic breakdown products from our bodies. Daily bowel movements ensure these toxins are swiftly removed. Conversely, if you're constipated or dehydrated, your body will attempt to reabsorb water from the stool back into the bloodstream, inadvertently bringing along toxins.

This recycling of toxins and hormones is a continual process that contributes significantly to your overall toxic load. If toxins are not cleared, it's just recycling throughout the body over and over again.

Therefore, one of the most impactful actions for your longevity is ensuring daily bowel movements, promoting efficient toxin elimination, and contributing to your overall wellness. This is a vital step in the ongoing journey of managing your health. The digestion lessons will impact this the most.

Check out the lesson on digestion to review the Bristol scale and learn all about poop.

## Action Steps

1. **Populate:** rotate high-quality specific strains of probiotics to maximize function and diversity. Take PRO-FLORA AI+ Monday to Friday and PRO-FLORA GI on Saturday and Sunday
2. **Nurture:** Feed the beneficial bacteria with quality prebiotic foods that are high in fiber. Eat at least 6 cups of fruit and vegetables a day. Biohack with adding FIBER PLUS and LOVE MY GREENS to your daily smoothie, soups, or sauces
3. **Dazzle:** make, buy, eat fermented foods such as sauerkraut, kimchi, kombucha daily
4. **Recipes:** Check out our recipe on how to make your own kimchi in the appendix. It's easy, delicious, makes a giant batch, and your microbiome will thank you for it. There is a companion recipe book of my favorite recipes to support the lessons in this book available.
5. **Digestion** must be optimal to fight infection at each step. Review the digestion lesson.
6. **Identify food allergens**: Review why **Certainty About Food** is a required lesson.
7. **Master your blood sugar:** Review the lesson for action steps there.
8. **Get data:** Once you do the above steps and still feel that infection is a culprit, seek out a functional medicine provider and get the correct data you need from a comprehensive stool analysis only available from a functional medicine provider. Only treat based on scientific data. Prevent reinfection by doing the above steps first—order matters.

Supplements mentioned are available at www.mymdshop.com

# LESSON 4:
## CERTAINTY ABOUT FOOD IS REQUIRED

Certainty about our food is required. Yet reactions to food are increasing and seemingly becoming more and more unpredictable and random. These reactions are part of an ever-growing long list of other reactions escalating at an alarming rate when we consume food. How many people will get bloated, gassy, intense pain, diarrhea, or constipation after eating? How about pain, headache, or brain fog? These seemingly random reactions are causing severe fear, anxiety, panic, and physical and social isolation. This is food trauma.

Trauma associated with eating can start early in childhood. How many of us were constantly reminded to finish our plates? No waste, right? How many experienced intense reactions to eating? Stories of babies with colic, childhood constipation, or the sudden aversion to certain foods once vomited show how our lives can be filled with bad experiences relating to food.

As we grow, these food traumas don't just fade away. Some people find themselves taking over-the-counter medications and avoiding more and more foods, while others just live with decades of heartburn, food feeling stuck, and nausea — following meals.

Many people find themselves designing their lives around restroom accessibility, constantly dreading what could and will happen.

Typically, the real reasons and the root causes remain undetermined. Negative blood work, imaging, and countless office visits later, people are diagnosed with terms as broad and vague as "irritable bowel syndrome." Lots of over-the-counter medications and prescriptions are prescribed to help control these symptoms. Eventually, they always get worse.

## My Own Journey with Food Reactions

I can recall my own journey. After the birth of my first child, I got mastitis, a breast infection, and took antibiotics. As a result, the antibiotic caused me to develop a super-resistant infection known as C. difficile. This is a relentless battle with mucousy chronic diarrhea, made worse by almost anything I ate. Every time I ate, I had to run to the bathroom. I got scared to eat and lost a ton of weight. The reason, I later realized, was not solely the infection. Unbeknownst to me, I had developed a gluten sensitivity triggered by the significant hormone shifts post-pregnancy.

While I continued to eat gluten regularly, my health declined, marked by fatigue, hair loss, and chronic pain. I was shocked nearly a decade later to discover that this deterioration was linked to my continued gluten consumption, which worsened digestive problems and other food allergies.

The most frustrating part of all this was my physicians' dismissal of these genuine symptoms. There were scientifically clear reasons for how the infection, my digestive issues, my food sensitivities, and my hormones were connected. I later found out I actually had genetic gluten sensitivity the whole time, but hormone changes just increased the reactions. More about gluten later.

Beyond the physical toll, food trauma has a huge social, emotional, and professional impact. They can limit our travel plans, social engagements, dining choices, and even if and how we work. People become hermits, socially isolated, or get used to saying "no" to everything. This leads to anxiety and depression. Fear becomes the default, and that's not living a life. That's suffering.

My experience and those of my patients of going to see doctors and specialists is traumatic. In their quest for clarity, some turn to allergists, only to be informed that their food reactions don't align with classic "allergies." If their testing is negative, it will make all of you who know your reactions are real feel like you're not believed or going crazy. Self-confidence is eroded, and frustration towards your doctors grows. I asked a room of 100 people how safe they felt with their doctor; the average number was 5/10. Interestingly, when I asked the medical providers in the group the same question, their numbers were even lower, 3/10. Isn't it ironic that those of us who work in the profession feel even more unsafe because we know it's factory medicine?

Some resort to gastrointestinal specialists and undergo procedures like endoscopies or colonoscopies, but the results are also "normal." These same individuals are often labeled with the now all-too-familiar term "irritable bowel syndrome." This isn't a diagnosis; it's a description of the symptoms. Try asking your gastrointestinal doctor if they believe food has anything to do with your symptoms; uniformly, you're told food doesn't matter. So, does that mean you're insane?

## Is Google or Elimination Diets the Answer?

Is the solution to go on Google or seek an alternative healthcare provider like a naturopathic physician? The first thing that happens is that most patients may be advised, without concrete testing, to embark on elimination diets. Such diets often entail cutting out broad food categories, sometimes encompassing 30 to 40 different foods. Whether diagnosed with a particular condition or simply seeking relief from unspecified symptoms, many are prescribed these diets. Specific protocols, such as the autoimmune protocol (AIP) diet, claim to address a range of autoimmune diseases by removing an extensive list of purported triggering foods. Other diets, like the Gut and Psychology Syndrome (GAPS) or fermentable oligosaccharides, disaccharides, monosaccharides, and polyols (FODMAP), are similarly recommended, while some individuals pivot entirely to vegetarian or vegan diets. Considerable shifts in your diet, eliminating huge categories of food abruptly, disrupt your gut and nutritional status.

Another huge problem is that elimination diets are inherently generalized and lack personalization. Patients might inadvertently deprive themselves of nutrient-dense foods in eliminating vast food categories. Also, by excluding certain foods, they may overcompensate by consuming larger quantities of other foods, potentially making things worse. This happens all the time. Somebody goes dairy-free. They don't get better. That's because they're now consuming vast quantities of almond milk, which they had no idea they were actually having the actual reaction to. A client, Julie, discovered through my program that it was vanilla in her almond milk and not even the dairy that was causing her IBS. She has been on eight years of elimination diet without improvement and was down to 98 pounds.

Some people get some immediate benefit from elimination diets. But they don't stay better and usually start to get worse as they consume more problematic foods they didn't know about. These diets, often misunderstood, were never intended as long-term solutions or generally applied to anyone who found them on Google. Being on extreme elimination diets is expensive, time-consuming, and socially isolating. If only it worked and solved problems long term.

There needs to be a science-rooted and data-driven solution to this problem. But where do we currently stand concerning data collection for understanding food reactions? Regrettably, our scope remains limited. Many patients approach allergists, undergoing skin or blood tests designed primarily to detect food allergies. This testing predominantly identifies IgE-mediated reactions, which are rapid and severe allergic responses. However, many symptoms, such as fatigue, hair loss, pain, insomnia, and anxiety, aren't caused by IgE allergies but are instead influenced by a diverse array of factors, including more subtle food allergies, sensitivities, digestive issues, and even infections.

This complexity makes accurate diagnosis challenging. Yet, patients who consult allergists often receive a skewed perspective, suggesting that allergist tests are the definitive solution. When these tests return inconclusive, patients are written off and left confused and frustrated. Few allergists refer these patients to functional medicine doctors because they don't believe that digestion has anything to do with it, and they claim that food sensitivities and intolerances are not real. This simply isn't true. Primary medical clinics and centers address food intolerances as real reactions and have various protocols trying to help people figure out what those are. Unfortunately, the testing of food sensitivities does present some challenges.

## Demystifying Food Sensitivities: Beyond Classic Allergies

Let's shift our focus to food sensitivities. Unlike the IgE-mediated allergic reactions we've discussed, sensitivities often relate to other immune allergic responses like IgG or IgA reactions.

## IgE (Immunoglobulin E): Fast Allergic Reactions (Minutes-Hours)

Function: IgE antibodies are primarily associated with allergic responses and defense against parasites. When your body encounters allergens like pollen or certain foods, it can trigger an allergic response. IgE antibodies play a central role in this process, causing the release of histamines and other chemicals that lead to allergic symptoms.

Location: IgE antibodies are found in relatively small amounts in the bloodstream and mucous membranes.

## IgG (Immunoglobulin G): Slow Allergic Reactions (Hours-Days)

Function: IgG antibodies are the most common type of antibody in the bloodstream and are vital for long-term immunity. They play a key role in fighting bacterial and viral infections. IgG antibodies can also cross the placenta during pregnancy, providing temporary immunity to the fetus.

Location: IgG antibodies are present in the bloodstream and are distributed throughout the body.

## IgA (Immunoglobulin A):
## Mucus Membrane Allergic Reactions

Function: IgA antibodies are essential for defending the mucosal surfaces of the body, such as the respiratory, gastrointestinal, and genitourinary tracts. They provide a first line of defense against pathogens like bacteria and viruses by preventing them from attaching to and invading the mucosal tissues.

Location: IgA antibodies are primarily found in mucous secretions, including saliva, tears, mucus, and breast milk. Secretory IgA in breast milk provides passive immunity to infants.

These IgG & IgA responses may be more insidious, causing nebulous symptoms that aren't necessarily gut-related. These delayed allergic responses and mucus membrane reactions can take even days for vague symptoms to show up.

Tragically, mainstream medicine trivializes these sensitivities, deeming them figments of an anxious person's imagination. However, they are merely different parts of our immune system, with slower and more ambiguous reactions. The delay in response or vagueness of these reactions complicates scientific studies. An example of this is that a classic allergy skin test creates very easy-to-read IgE-mediated immediate allergic responses clearly visible on the skin. IgG-mediated reactions often can take 4-10 days to show a reaction, and it's nowhere near the induration (thickening and hardening of soft tissues) visible as the immediate reactions. These IgG allergic reactions are not measured by the allergist. They are dismissed.

Additionally, these slower sensitivities-type allergic reactions can produce symptoms like fatigue, headache, abdominal pain, diarrhea, and symptoms that allergists don't deem to be allergic. However, those who've experienced a known reaction to something know that eating certain foods can cause you pain. Well, in the world of the allergist, it can't be. Do you trust your body and the data and reactions it's giving you, or do you believe the allergist who says it can't possibly happen? I'd put my money and trust in my own body, and I trust you, the person experiencing it.

Medical doctors' skepticism around accurate tests for food sensitivities isn't entirely unfounded. Numerous companies market food sensitivity tests, many of which have garnered a reputation for their questionable quality and accuracy. Having personally tested thousands of patients using over 20 different tests, I can attest that many of these tests lack validity. A multitude of factors contribute to this. For one, the inherent vagueness, delay, and individual variability in reactions make them challenging to study. Furthermore, the source material used for testing, known as the antigen source, isn't always pure, isolated, or accurate. This compromises the credibility of the results.

The population of people who have food reactions already have altered immune systems in some way; this can lead to false positives or false negatives. In essence, a person might not actually react to a particular food item, but the test might indicate otherwise due to their irregular immune system. They may have a higher rate of error in their test results.

However, it's crucial to note that not all tests are unusable. A few companies have developed high-quality tests, although they remain in the minority. A commonly used test favored by many functional medicine doctors is not only pricey but, based on my experience and that of many providers, highly inaccurate. It's not uncommon for this test, along with several others, to indicate positive reactions for 30-50% of the food items tested. This can lead patients down a rabbit hole of expensive, time-consuming, and nutrient-depleting elimination diets. They often find no actual reaction when they eventually reintroduce or inadvertently consume these foods.

It's precisely experiences like these that fuel skepticism among medical professionals. Faced with the unreliable nature of many tests, they might discourage patients from enjoying food. A critical component of the Food Mapping System is its emphasis on the significance of negative test results. Often, individuals anticipate their results to highlight a multitude of food sensitivities, only to discover that only a few or even no foods are causing their reactions.

These negative results can be more informative than finding a long list of positive foods. Such results accentuate that what isn't causing a reaction can sometimes be more enlightening than what is. This "ruling out" process is essential because it encourages patients and practitioners to adopt a more curious and investigative approach. I call this my mantra:

*"What it isn't is even more important than what it is."*

If a person displays a multitude of symptoms but tests negative for food sensitivities and allergies, it begs the most curious question. What else could it be if it isn't what I assumed to be an allergic food reaction? The answers can range from digestive issues and infections to non-allergic food reactions. Someone could be reacting to a specific pesticide used on certain crops or have a chemical sensitivity to a naturally occurring substance in a group of plants. It's not always about allergies, and understanding these layers is crucial for interpreting even the most accurate test results. Most of the time, digestion plays a huge role in the reactions to food rather than allergies. This was explored in the lesson on why digestion is the holy grail in understanding food-related reactions.

One of the most poignant lessons from my experiences is that food reactions aren't exclusive to gut-related issues. Symptoms like chronic TMJ pain in the jaw or neuropathy, leading to numbness and tingling in the limbs, can often be traced back to reactions from food items such as gluten, dairy, or even vanilla or sesame seeds! With the right diagnostic system and accurate testing, one can pinpoint whether a reaction is allergy-related, stems from a digestive or infectious issue, or arises from a chemical sensitivity. For example, Jennifer, who had chronic regional pain syndrome, found out it was eggs, just eggs for her. Her symptoms are already 50% less in the past two months.

I created the Food Mapping System from the need to validate and address people's genuine reactions to food scientifically. However, tackling this complex issue is more than just a solitary journey. There isn't a singular test or doctor with all the answers. The system was designed to address a range of health issues, from irritable bowel syndrome and chronic heartburn to harder-to-treat conditions like mast cell activation or histamine intolerance. Even diagnoses seemingly unrelated to food, such as fibromyalgia or POTS, Lupus can find clarity through this system. It's been a curious and fascinating journey to see how no matter what someone's diagnosis is or whether or not they have one, undergoing the Food Mapping System to digest, test, learn, and discern with guidance is the key to success. This doesn't exist, and I had to create it. I have a beautifully accurate reproducible system for determining someone's food reactions. It isn't a simple one-pill or one-test answer. It's a scientific method that requires your data, education, and guidance in the system. That's my best answer, and I'm happy to report it's a darn good one.

There are hundreds of video case studies of people who've gone through the Food Mapping System I developed. My point and the biggest lesson here is that food reactions are real. You are seen.

You are heard. You are believed. Most importantly, I know with 100% certainty that a system exists to get you out. With an open, curious mind, learn more about the Food Mapping System I created.

## What About Gluten?

"Should I avoid gluten?" This is a question I frequently encounter, and it's undoubtedly on the minds of many individuals keen on optimizing their health.

I won't assert that gluten is universally harmful, nor am I here to claim that it is problematic for everyone. The reality, however, is nuanced. A significant number of people do struggle with gluten, and understanding its potential effects is more intricate than it might seem at first glance.

Let's embark on a journey of understanding, where I present the scientific rationale behind considering a temporary hiatus from gluten – perhaps for six months. Why such a specific timeframe? Let's unpack that.

In the past decade, the discourse around gluten intolerance has seen a dramatic shift. What was once perceived as a benign element in our diet has, for some, emerged as a potential adversary. Through this chapter, we aim to demystify the genuine medical concerns surrounding gluten intolerance and offer insights into the intricate nature of diagnosing this condition. Let's delve deeper into the gluten puzzle and arm ourselves with knowledge for more informed dietary choices.

# The Rise Of Gluten Intolerance

Gluten intolerance, sometimes referred to as non-celiac gluten sensitivity (NCGS), has firmly established its presence as a medical fact. Many scientific and medical institutions, including the Mayo Clinic, recognize it as a distinct medical condition from other forms of gluten reaction or allergy. Individuals experiencing symptoms such as gastrointestinal distress, fatigue, brain fog, and headaches after consuming gluten-rich foods have raised their voices, asserting that something is amiss. For them, gluten intolerance is not a figment of imagination but a daily reality. Nobody believes them, yet they know it's real for them. Note many of the symptoms above have nothing to do with the gut.

**Here's a Short List of Symptoms of Gluten Intolerance:**

Gastrointestinal Symptoms:
- Abdominal pain
- Bloating
- Diarrhea
- Constipation
- Nausea
- Vomiting
- Gas or flatulence
- Acid reflux or heartburn
- Acid reflux or heartburn
- Cramping
- Crohn's & Ulcerative colitis
- Irritable bowel syndrome

Neurological and Psychological Symptoms:
- Headaches
- Mood swings
- Dementia
- Migraines
- ADD
- Tinnitus
- Brain fog or cognitive impairment
- Irritability
- Vertigo
- Anxiety
- POTS (Postural Orthostatic Tachycardia)
- Fatigue
- Depression
- Multiple sclerosis
- Dysautonomia

Skin Symptoms:
- Dermatitis herpetiformis (a skin rash associated with celiac disease)
- Eczema
- Itchy skin
- Psoriasis
- Lichen Sclerosus
- Rosacea

Musculoskeletal Symptoms:

- Joint pain
- Muscle pain
- Muscle weakness
- Osteoporosis or low bone density
- Rheumatoid arthritis
- Fibromyalgia
- Mixed Connective Tissue Disorders

Miscellaneous Symptoms:

- Fatigue or weakness
- Anemia (iron deficiency)
- Mouth ulcers or canker sores
- Weight loss (unintentional)
- Weight gain (less common, but it can occur)
- Autoimmune disease of every kind

It's important to note that the severity and combination of symptoms can vary widely among individuals with gluten-related disorders. Some individuals may experience multiple symptoms, while others may have only one or two. Additionally, some people may have atypical or silent forms of these conditions, meaning they experience minimal or no digestive symptoms.

# The Testing Quandary

Unraveling the complexities of gluten intolerance hinges on accurate and consistent testing. But herein lies a significant hurdle. While celiac disease, a severe autoimmune condition, stands as the primary benchmark for diagnosing gluten-related disorders, it's not without its challenges. A diagnosis typically involves blood tests, with a subsequent intestinal biopsy for confirmation.

However, a large portion of individuals with gluten intolerance don't fit the celiac profile. The waters are further muddied when it comes to establishing a definitive diagnosis for celiac disease. Some gastrointestinal specialists believe a colon biopsy revealing damage from the autoimmune response is the answer. But what about patients who exhibit clear indicators of celiac disease through blood work or genetic assessments but have a biopsy that doesn't show the end-stage damage? There's an ongoing debate within the medical community, with some advocating that the benchmark for diagnosis shouldn't rely solely on the severe outcomes of untreated celiac disease. Such a narrow viewpoint is limiting and can lead to misdiagnosis.

To address these gaps, both medical professionals and patients need to be well-versed in the range of available blood and genetic tests. Incorporating family history into the diagnosis process is also crucial.

Now, let's consider another layer of this intricate puzzle. Imagine an individual suspecting a gluten-related issue, yet all their celiac tests come back negative. The immediate assumption is that it's a psychological manifestation. However, recent shifts in the medical community acknowledge a substantial number of individuals who genuinely react to gluten without being celiac patients. A classic example involves individuals with an IgE or an immediate allergic reaction to gluten or wheat. Symptoms can range from tongue swelling to breathlessness upon gluten ingestion. These immediate reactions, coupled with allergist tests, can quickly pinpoint an IgE-mediated allergic reaction. While these individuals aren't celiac patients, they certainly shouldn't consume gluten.

On the other hand, there are those who experience severe symptoms, but neither fit the celiac diagnosis nor test positive for IgE. Here, we stumble upon the celiac vs. non-celiac vs. IgE allergic dilemma. Might there be others with varying reactions to gluten, such as the IgG-mediated delayed reactions or the IgA-mediated mucus membrane responses?

The concept of non-celiac gluten sensitivity (NCGS) has been a contentious topic within the medical realm. A significant challenge in diagnosing NCGS is the absence of specific markers or tests, unlike celiac disease. Those suspected of having NCGS often find standard celiac tests, like serology and biopsies, returning negative results. This discrepancy between the symptoms and the test results adds to the frustration for those grappling with genuine gluten intolerance.

Often, their IgE tests from allergists come back negative. As highlighted before, the reliability of IgG and IgA tests currently available is questionable, compounded by a lack of training for providers to discern and interpret accurate tests.

## Food Mapping Emerges as Fast Pass

With a lack of proper testing of gluten sensitivity from IgG and IgA, people with symptoms are left to fend for themselves or labeled as crazy. This question can be answered with reliable testing through Food Mapping and working with Transform. We detail and explore all the testing and questions that people have about gluten. The fact is, most of the people we work with find out that they have some sort of reaction to gluten. Having a better understanding of all the different kinds of testing and your own results is a powerful guide. We've been accurately identifying gluten sensitivity not only in those we work with, but their better understanding of genetics has identified these problems in at least three generations of people in their family. Our testing and training allow people to experience their generational impact on accurately identifying gluten and other food intolerances.

Once they feel better and understand their data, it becomes a powerful tool for the children, siblings, and parents. The most significant action one can take is to learn more about working with us to experience the Food Mapping System.

**Take a pause from gluten.** In light of the challenges in pinning down a reliable diagnostic test for gluten intolerance, many are tempted to embrace broad-spectrum elimination diets, sidelining vast categories of food. I'm against such drastic, broad stroke measures for a variety of reasons. However, given the ubiquitous nature of gluten intolerance and the intricacies surrounding its diagnosis, I do advocate for a measured approach.

For those grappling with the symptoms I've detailed, a three-month hiatus from gluten can be insightful. This means a complete commitment to a gluten-free regimen. If this sounds daunting or not feasible at the present moment, then it might not be the right choice for you. Should you seek concrete Food Mapping insights and guidance to discern whether this step is necessary for your health journey, we're here to assist. But when it comes to food trials and understanding your body's reactions, gluten should be at the top of your list.

**Empowering the individual is key.** Imagine this: If you were told there's over a 50% chance that gluten might be the cause of one of your health symptoms, would you want to uncover the truth? Would you be motivated to potentially change the trajectory of that ailment?

Research highlights the many ways gluten interacts with and affects our immune systems. Interestingly, our body's immune response to gluten can last for up to six months.

Given the challenges with current testing methods, a straightforward approach for many is to eliminate gluten entirely for three months. Pay attention to any changes during this phase. Afterward, reintroducing gluten and observing your body's reaction can offer critical insights. After such a detox phase, any adverse reactions upon reintroduction often become significantly more pronounced, indicating possible intolerance.

When navigating the complexities of gluten intolerance and its broad health implications, one message stands out: the importance of personal agency. Those suspecting gluten intolerance should collaborate closely with health professionals, understand the intricacies of testing, and, when deemed appropriate, consider a three-month gluten-free trial. This journey is not just about health but about individuals actively participating in their well-being and championing their own bodies.

At the time of the publishing of this edition, we are excited to begin to offer our Food Mapping System for anyone who wants 100% clarity on their food reactions. There's more to come, and depending on the time you read this, you may be getting on a waiting list or be able to sign up to work with us directly.

## Action Steps

1. Do not order any self-order test kits for food sensitivities; they really are inaccurate.
2. Do not go on another broad brush stroke elimination diet.
3. Do eliminate gluten for three months if you have any of the symptoms I've highlighted in this chapter for gluten intolerance.
4. Make sure they understand digestion. Many symptoms from broken steps in digestion are erroneously blamed on food allergies.
5. Watch the many videos on our YouTube channel about the Food Mapping System and how education, direct medical guidance, and accurate data have restored people's freedom and lives.
6. Fast pass your confusion around gluten by working with us on Food Mapping to help not just you but three generations of your family at the same time because… psst, it's genetic.
7. Psst… here's a secret. Check out [www.MYFoodMapping.com](www.MYFoodMapping.com)

# LESSON 5:
# BLOOD SUGAR MASTERY

There are specific symptoms and diagnoses that, over the past decade, scream of blood sugar as the root cause. I'd like you to meet Kristen and see if you can guess or pinpoint what symptoms jump out at me as being blood sugar swings triggered. You will learn throughout this chapter what are the tell-tale signs.

*Meet Kristen, a lactation consultant struggling with Sjögren's, Lupus, and chronic fatigue for 15+ years. She thought that blood sugar was the least likely problem she would have as a healthcare professional. After all, she doesn't have diabetes (typically the only problem doctors focus on).*

*Over the years, she developed a laundry list of symptoms that left her without a clear diagnosis or answers. Her doctors called it idiopathic, meaning they didn't know why. She had severe insomnia, hot flashes, irritability, weight gain, hair loss, chronic joint pain, headaches, brain fog, anxiety, and gastroparesis (her bowels didn't move food well). She also had trouble swallowing, which was one of the scariest and newest symptoms. She saw multiple specialists, including many gastrointestinal doctors, rheumatologists, neurologists, psychologists, and gynecologists. After taking a long list of medications and invasive procedures, including many endoscopies and colonoscopies, she still had no answers and no relief.*

*She was a successful medical professional, but her focus, brain fog, and growing insecurity around her own abilities* to improve her symptoms were taking a toll. Her husband and her teenagers were as worried about her as she was. Something had to be done differently. Something had to be done outside the system she was trained and worked in.

She was one of the first clients who found us through social media and reached out to work with us nearly eight years ago. In the first few weeks, as she was going through the blood sugar modules, she started making changes to how and when she ate. As a medical professional who worked with new moms and their ability to breastfeed their babies, she counseled them on proper nutrition and hydration. She could have had resistance to learning something new about blood sugar. But, to Kristen's credit, her superpower is that she's an eager learner and an even better implementor.

While watching the video training on how to balance blood sugar throughout the day and in working with our functional nutritionist, she started with eating within 30 minutes of waking up and ending the day with a cup of warm Golden Balance with some additional collagen in it.

To her surprise, after just the first two weeks, her headaches were gone. She had these at least ten times a month! Shockingly, that wasn't it; soon after, she found herself sleeping for the first time in three years, the whole night! Over the next month, her joint pain nearly all but disappeared. By three months, her swallowing improved, as well as her pain.

Today, eight years later, Kristen has lost weight. She's pain-free, exercising. Her kids had joined her in learning and implementing during the program, and there has been a massive shift in the health of her husband and children. They're traveling, and Kristen is working at her full capacity as a lactation consultant. She's been on multiple interviews on social media, sharing her newfound knowledge and results.

Like Kristen, most people have no idea that there were clear signs all along that her symptoms were related to an underlying problem with how her body handles blood sugar. Like all conventionally trained medical professionals, if someone does not have diabetes (having met the laboratory criteria for having frequent high blood sugars most of the time), then there must not be a blood sugar problem.

A common misconception regarding the HbA1c blood test: many individuals and doctors believe that a typical result implies stable and healthy blood sugar levels. The HbA1c test indeed provides an average blood sugar level over the past three months, assisting in diagnosing chronic high blood sugar and diabetes.
However, it falls short of identifying issues of low blood sugar or frequent fluctuations between high and low levels, which can be the root of various symptoms.

This is a huge blind spot. Blood sugar mastery isn't about whether or not you have diabetes. Many of Kristen's and perhaps even your symptoms have to do with the swings in blood sugar from high to low or vice versa. Many of her symptoms had to do with low blood sugar episodes.

Let's dive into a preview. Arm yourself with a highlighter and take note of specific symptoms in Kristen's story that immediately stood out to me as related to blood sugar swings. Soon, you'll recognize them, too.

As you proceed through this chapter, keep a keen eye on why these symptoms are often misunderstood and not typically associated with blood sugar levels:

- Headaches
- Insomnia
- Hot Flashes
- Anxiety
- Irritability
- Weight Gain
- Pain
- Brain Fog
- Gastroparesis (difficulty moving food through the bowels)
- Autoimmune diseases such as Lupus and Sjögren's

Highlight these symptoms and maintain attentiveness to their often-overlooked connection to blood sugar throughout this chapter.

I chose Kristen's story as most of her symptoms are classic for blood sugar swings and low blood sugar. You will see how this all ties together. Perhaps you are starting to see some of your own symptoms? Have you been tested for diabetes and told you don't have it? Do you now question your doctor's bias and perhaps your own around the role of blood sugar? You should. Let's get out of the box on this.

# The New Concept Is Blood Sugar SWINGS As The Main Problem

Understanding blood sugar isn't just about recognizing high levels or diagnosing diabetes. The real concern is the rapid swings in blood sugar levels, which many might overlook. Surprisingly, these fluctuations can manifest in myriad ways, often leading to misdiagnoses or being brushed off as complex, unexplained symptoms.

Consider this: When you enjoy a meal, it's not just about satisfying hunger. As you eat, a complex process unfolds inside your body. Digestive enzymes and stomach acids work diligently, breaking down your food into microscopic components. This food predominantly contains fats, proteins, and carbohydrates. It's the carbohydrates, when digested, that convert into glucose, causing a surge in blood sugar levels.

This is where the pancreas springs into action. Located near the stomach, this organ vigilantly monitors blood sugar levels. A substantial carbohydrate intake can cause a rapid rise in these levels. Acting as the body's gatekeeper, the pancreas releases insulin to counteract this surge, ensuring blood sugar remains within an optimal range.

Insulin is not just any hormone; it's the maestro of blood sugar regulation. It facilitates the uptake of sugar by various tissues. Any excess sugar is then stored for future use. The primary goal of insulin is to reduce blood sugar swiftly and efficiently.

The detailed diagram illustrates insulin's numerous functions, highlighting how it manages sugar distribution and storage in the body. But what happens when one consistently consumes a carbohydrate-rich diet? The pancreas goes into overdrive, releasing excessive insulin. Such frequent insulin activity can cause blood sugar levels to plummet several times a day.

Hypoglycemia, or low blood sugar, can manifest in myriad ways. While we'll explore its symptoms in detail later, it's crucial to realize that the problem isn't merely high blood sugar. Instead, it's the dramatic shifts, the highs and lows, that trigger various symptoms for people everywhere.

Instead of viewing blood sugar levels as a simple high or low issue, imagine it as an oscillating wave. This wave-like behavior illustrates the body's non-binary nature – it's not just about 'yes' or 'no.' In fact, understanding the amplitude of these waves, their peaks and troughs, and the rate of these fluctuations is crucial.

## Insulin and Glucagon

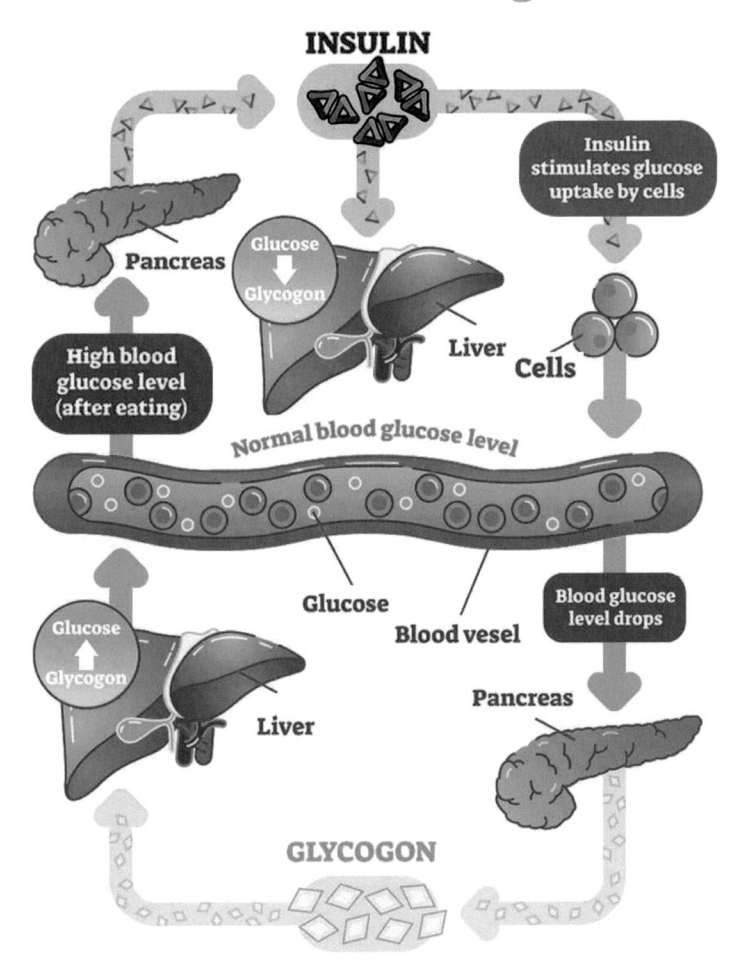

**INSULIN**

- Insulin stimulates glucose uptake by cells
- Pancreas
- Glucose → Glycogen
- Liver
- Cells
- High blood glucose level (after eating)
- Normal blood glucose level
- Glucose
- Blood vesel
- Glucose ← Glycogen
- Liver
- Blood glucose level drops
- Pancreas

**GLYCOGON**

## Blood Sugar Chart

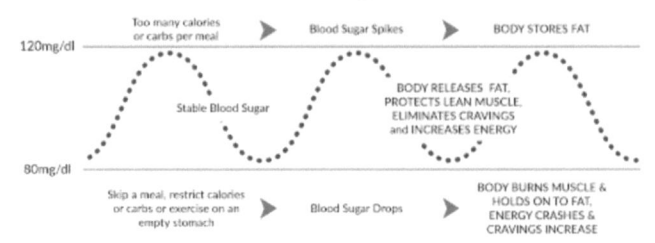

Fig. An example of blood sugar levels cycling throughout the day

The figure above illustrates these fluctuations. While it provides a reference point, remember everyone's optimal range varies. Some might feel the effects of low blood sugar at 80, while for others, it could be 50. It's less about the exact numbers and more about recognizing these continuous shifts.

Interestingly, genetics can influence the magnitude of these swings. Some individuals experience broader fluctuations, reaching higher peaks. This can be indicative of conditions like diabetes or even polycystic ovarian syndrome (PCOS) - a condition that often eludes proper diagnosis. For instance, Jane's blood sugar might shoot up to 250 after a soda, while Caitlin's might only reach 120. Such dramatic spikes prompt the pancreas to release copious amounts of insulin, which then pushes the blood sugar down sharply.

You don't have to be diabetic to experience this. Most people may not qualify as diabetic, but they still grapple with substantial blood sugar fluctuations throughout the day.

One of the primary diagnostic tools for blood sugar issues is the HbA1c test. However, it mainly determines average blood sugar levels over three months. It doesn't offer insights into daily fluctuations. So, while your doctor might declare you free from diabetes based on the HbA1c, it doesn't necessarily mean you're free from blood sugar issues. The core issue might be the rapid swings in your blood sugar levels, resulting in a plethora of symptoms. It's vital to shift the conversation from just high blood sugar to understanding and managing these daily fluctuations.

## Low Blood Sugar is a Real Devil

When discussing low blood sugar, what definitions spring to mind? And where might we be getting it wrong?

Contrary to popular belief, low blood sugar doesn't solely manifest as nausea, dizziness, or a light headache. Those with diabetes, due to their insulin treatments, often experience pronounced episodes of low blood sugar characterized by feelings of faintness, excessive sweating, and palpitations.

### Hypoglycemia
(low blood sugar)

- Belly growling, nausea, stomach upset
- Heart palpitations
- Sweating
- Dizziness, POTS, vertigo
- Shakiness, tremors, restless leg, leg cramps
- Pain flares
- Headaches, migraines
- Sleepiness, insomnia, fatigue
- Irritability, "hangry"
- Confusion, brain fog, dementia
- Anxiety, depression, ADD/ADHD
- Hormone imbalance

These severe episodes, often associated with diabetes, have become the hallmark symptoms of hypoglycemia. While these are valid and "classic" symptoms, they don't paint the entire picture, as depicted in the image above.

Indeed, low blood sugar isn't exclusive to people with diabetes. The average individual also encounters these episodes, albeit subtly.

While they might not experience dramatic symptoms like fainting or sweating, the signs can be discreet yet identifiable once you recognize the pattern. These nuanced episodes often go unnoticed, sidelining a significant health issue regardless of one's diabetic condition.

But what causes these less conventional symptoms of hypoglycemia? A sudden dip from high to low blood sugar sets off alarm bells in the body. It interprets this fluctuation as a threat, prompting a cascade of responses from vital organs. This perceived danger sends muscles into overdrive, the heart beats faster, and the hormone-producing adrenal glands go on high alert. Elevated levels of cortisol and adrenaline, resulting from these frequent low blood sugar episodes, disrupt the body's natural rhythms, putting standard functions like digestion and hormone regulation on pause.

This fight or flight state due to persistent low blood sugar can wreak havoc on one's mental and physical well-being. Elevated hormones from adrenal glands and the brain, such as norepinephrine and epinephrine, can induce feelings of irritability, anxiety, and a lack of focus.

Despite these evident links, mental health professionals seldom attribute such symptoms to regular blood sugar fluctuations.

Additionally, sustained high cortisol levels may lead to weight gain, chronic pain, and persistent fatigue.

As you'll discover later in this chapter, various hormonal imbalances stem from these blood sugar swings, impacting daily life in myriad ways. Consider Kristen's experience as an example: stabilizing her daily blood sugar levels was instrumental in mitigating her symptoms.

The key takeaway? Low blood sugar is more deceptive than it appears. It doesn't always manifest as medically-defined hypoglycemia. Throughout your day, subtle symptoms may signal underlying blood sugar issues. This revelation often proves enlightening for many of my clients. For instance: morning nausea, heightened anxiety during the night, or frequent afternoon energy crashes can all point to this underlying issue.

Symptoms such as these, seemingly unrelated to meals, are often indicative of a day spent in a flux of high and low blood sugar. Observing daily patterns and symptoms can offer insights into an individual's blood sugar stability—the tell-tale signs, though sometimes tough to discern, never lie.

While we've touched upon some signals to watch out for, we'll dive deeper into the most overlooked indicators of blood sugar swings later in this chapter.

## What is Blood Sugar Mastery?

**Balance your macronutrients.** This is the first and most important building block of blood sugar mastery. Too often, people are on heart-healthy diets or various elimination diets that decrease the amount of protein and especially fat in their diet. It is as simple as taking a look at your plate and seeing: is there fat, protein, and fiber on my plate equally?

**Fat got a bad rap.** Most people think about fat, and they think about weight gain and elevated cholesterol. However, fat is essential. That's why many fats provide healthy essential fatty acids. Fats we eat are digested to become the fatty acids that are the building and repair blocks our bodies need. Did you know that hormones are made from fatty acids? Unless you eat a balanced amount of fat, you struggle to make needed hormones like insulin, human growth hormone, estrogen, and testosterone.

The other function that fat has is that it takes a lot of digestive steps and time to turn into glucose, i.e., sugar. So, it slowly and steadily releases blood sugar. In that sense, it can ground your carbohydrates. Meaning it's the form of glucose that becomes slow-release in your meal, making blood sugar stabilization and mastery throughout the day much more manageable. It's a slow up and down, unlike simply eating sugar or bread that turns rapidly into sugar, causing spikes.

This is also why taking omega-3 fatty acids is critical. These fats, from mostly fish sources or algae, help you make healthy hormones. Also, did you know that your nerves and your brain are mostly fat? 60% of the human brain is fat. So how can someone repair brain cells or nerve cells if they don't eat fat? They cannot. This is why eating fat is critical to blood sugar mastery throughout the day, but it also has many other benefits that will be discussed in multiple lessons. This is also why I recommend the intake of omega-3 in the action steps and the eating of fats from healthy sources. Examples of healthy sources of fat are:

| Oils from small fatty fish are key | Avoid large predator fish | Sustainable choices that are high in omegas |
|---|---|---|
| • Sardines<br>• Anchovies<br>• Mackerel<br>• Wild salmon | • Full of mercury and toxins collected from their prey<br>• Avoid<br>   ○ Shark<br>   ○ Tuna<br>   ○ Halibut<br>   ○ Swordfish | • Shrimp<br>• Crab<br>• Shellfish<br>• Oysters<br>• Mussels<br>• Clams<br>• Squid |

- Small fatty fish like wild-caught salmon, sardines, mackerel, and anchovies are high in omega 3s, and they do not prey on many other small fish. Predator fish, who mainly eat other fish, concentrate pesticides and toxins from their prey.
- Avocados
- Coconut oil
- Ghee (clarified butter)
- Olive Oil
- Nuts and seeds

Proteins help stabilize blood sugar. These complex molecules consist of amino acids found in all living organisms, including plants. Proteins and their breakdown into amino acids play numerous critical roles in the body, carrying out most cellular work. Despite their essential role, some individuals avoid a balanced protein diet due to concerns about fat or dietary choices such as vegetarianism or veganism. Nevertheless, you can still get lots of protein from plant sources. The unique characteristic of proteins is their slow digestion and breakdown into amino acids and glucose, ensuring a gradual conversion into glucose. This slow conversion helps maintain stable blood sugar levels, preventing sudden spikes or drops and should constitute a significant portion of your dietary intake, as illustrated below.

What are excellent sources of protein?

- Land: Beef, chicken, pork, lamb, game, eggs (preferably organic or grass-fed)
- Sea: Fatty smaller fish such as salmon, mackerel, sardines, shrimp, shellfish, and squid (wild preferred over farmed)
- Plants: Beans, tempeh (fermented soy), tofu (organic)

**Carbohydrates** are foods that are primarily composed of sugars, starch, and cellulose. They break down into glucose but at a much more direct and faster rate than protein or fat. Therefore, when filling your plate with a third carbohydrate, you need to consider the following concepts. Pick carbohydrates that are high in cellulose (fiber) and low in sugar or starches. Why? Starches and sugars quickly turn into glucose, causing blood sugar spikes. Foods that are high in carbohydrates that are high in fiber or cellulose content take longer to digest and turn into glucose or sugar.

The principle is to avoid simple carbohydrates that are low in fiber, such as flour, bread, pasta, or white rice. Opt to limit 'white' foods as much as possible due to their processing, which depletes them of significant fiber and nutrients. So when eating grains, strive for brown whole grains, their original color. Instead of grains or whites being the third on your plate, go for the greens and colors of plants.

Think avocados, cabbage, cauliflower, cucumbers, vegetables. Think zucchini noodles over flour noodles. A third of the plate as vegetables rather than grains is my own preference due to the power of fiber and plants and their impact on health and blood sugar.

What is an out-of-the-box way to slow down the carbohydrate release of glucose into the bloodstream? What if there's something you can add to your carbohydrate, let's say rice, that even if you eat it, you can slow the rate it releases into the blood, therefore reducing the insulin surge? Here's a little-known hack.

- Eat carbs last in the order of your meal. Let the protein and fat go first. This already lets the fat and protein get digested first, and they turn into glucose much more slowly. End your meal with rice, pasta, or potato if you're going to have them.

Do not start the meal with them first. Don't order the french fry as your appetizer at a restaurant. Instead go for the buffalo wings, steak bites, or hummus with vegetables.

- Add lemon juice, apple cider vinegar, or a product like DIGEST-IT that contains acid to your carbs to slow the release of glucose into the bloodstream. Make sure each meal contains a squeeze of lemon juice. Add apple cider vinegar to your soups. When making a sauce for anything, consider adding lemon or something acidic to it. Think lemon butter sauce. Even if you're eating a bowl of noodles, which is all carbohydrates, add apple cider vinegar or a squeeze of lemon to the broth. This will slow the release of glucose, lowering the spikes in blood sugar.

**How do you balance your plate?** Fat, protein, and fiber are essential nutrients in large quantities to make energy. One way to achieve this is by dividing your plate into thirds for each meal and snack: one-third for fat, one-third for protein, and one-third for fiber. This approach helps stabilize blood sugar levels since fat and protein provide a steady energy source for hours. Regarding fiber, prioritizing fiber-based carbohydrates such as leafy green vegetables, beans, and low-glycemic fruits is essential over simple carbohydrates like grains and processed foods.

I prefer to avoid counting calories or analyzing spreadsheets, so I designed a simple system that focuses on a simple idea like balancing your fat, fiber, and protein.

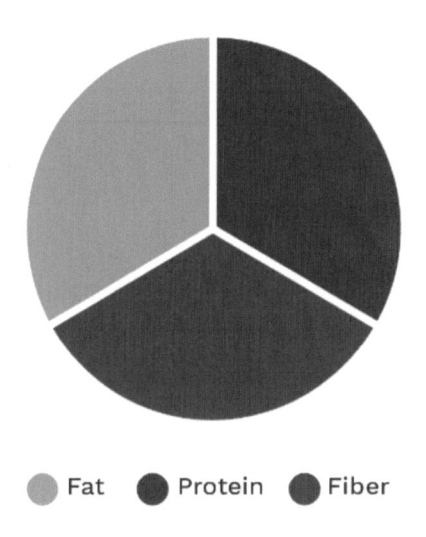

● Fat  ● Protein  ● Fiber

People often need to realize which fats, proteins, and fibers are high quality. Unhealthy fats, such as those in deep-fried and processed foods, are the enemy. Many healthy fats are critical for brain, hormones, and nerve health. Some excellent examples are organic butter, high-fat fish like mackerel and salmon, and organic pasture-raised beef, chicken, and pork. Vegetarian fat sources include avocados, nuts, olives, and MCT coconut oil.

There are many protein sources, including vegan options, that people need to eat more of. Animal protein sources include grass-fed beef, chicken, pork, and wild-caught fish. Vegans, in particular, struggle to get enough healthy fat and protein, which can lead to health problems. Beer and french fries are vegan but don't contain much healthy fat, protein, or fiber.

Some great vegan protein options include organic tofu, tempeh, seitan beans, spirulina, soy or pea protein crumbles, nutritional yeast, and protein pasta, to list a few. Some vegetarians occasionally eat fish to ensure they get the healthy omega-3s that are very difficult to get in high doses from plant sources.

**Bookending saves the day.** There are some pivotal ways in which we help people we work with to maintain a healthy blood sugar-balancing diet throughout the day. Through people writing down what they eat over 48 hours and a review with us, we ensure that they consume fat, protein, and fiber in their meals and snacks. If you do nothing else, doing the critical bookending the day every day would yield immediate results. This is the most important takeaway from this chapter.

I now want to share with you the number one mistake many people make in the morning - skipping breakfast. While some may say they're not hungry or feel nauseous, the real reason is often low blood sugar.
This can be prevented by eating a small snack before bed and having a balanced breakfast when you wake up. In fact, regularly eating throughout the day is essential to keeping your blood sugar levels stable. So, prioritize eating breakfast and maintaining a regular meal schedule to avoid these symptoms and keep your blood sugar in check.

People tend to overcomplicate breakfast and make it more difficult than it needs to be. One of the most significant objections is the lack of hunger or even feeling nauseated in the morning. However, it's essential to understand that low blood sugar can cause nausea, which your brain interprets as a signal to avoid eating or feeling not hungry. In reality, the opposite is true.

Having breakfast every morning as soon as possible is crucial for both adults and children to kickstart their metabolism, stimulate hormone production, and activate the liver's detoxification process. It plays a vital role in setting the right foundation for the day.

However, we need to approach breakfast differently. It's time to ditch the typical options like cereal, toast, or muffins. Why? These classic carbohydrate-based breakfasts lead to a significant spike in blood sugar, followed by a sharp drop, resulting in low blood sugar later on. Instead, let's start considering alternatives that include protein, fat, and fiber.

Think about incorporating eggs, breakfast meats, or preparing frittatas or quiches in advance so they only require a minute to warm up. Protein, fat, and fiber can be incredibly easy and convenient without compromising your health. Have you considered trying overnight chia pudding? It doesn't require cooking or heating and can be a nutritious option. It's time to let go of the usual breakfast items and focus on pre-planning meals that prioritize protein, fat, and fiber.

The possibilities for achieving better health and longevity are limitless. And the best part is that you'll notice immediate results.

Bookending your day with food is crucial for maintaining stable blood sugar levels. Eating a small snack before bed can prevent low blood sugar levels in the morning and keep you stable overnight. Many times, if you're unable to consume fiber, it's still beneficial to consume some fat and protein before bed. In this book, we have included a recipe for a fat bomb that I absolutely adore making. It contains various beneficial fats and proteins from nut butter, making it a perfect bedtime snack. If you want to add fiber, pair it with vegetable sticks.

And because some people don't like to eat before bed? Drink it! You don't want to drink something with high volume because you don't want to pee all night. So, you want to drink about six ounces or less of something like GOLDEN BALANCE. GOLDEN BALANCE is the most effective way to drink your fat and protein.

**GOLDEN BALANCE** is a delicious powerhouse of nutrient goodness that is a perfect addition to your bedtime routine.

- Highly Bioavailable Curcumin and Grass-Fed† Collagen Peptides

- If you consistently wake up between the hours of 2 and 4 a.m., consuming good fats and protein before bed can help to regulate fluctuating blood sugar levels that are contributing to this middle-of-the-night sleep disturbance. GOLDEN BALANCE contains anti-inflammatory, hormone, and blood sugar-balancing properties that will assist in keeping blood sugars stable so that you can sleep soundly through the night. This will allow your body to initiate all the vital restorative processes that contribute to optimum health.

- It starts with protein with medical-grade complete collagen in it. It's got coconut milk with the fat, and you can add any milk or cream in there for additional fat. Plus, herbs are the perfect blend for blood sugar balancing. Why not add powerful bioactive herbs to help stabilize blood sugar all night? Finally, make it taste delicious. My clients often call GOLDEN BALANCE a "hug in a mug."

Turmeric and curcumin are great for activating the liver to balance blood sugar and break down hormones. Adding that to your evening meal or drink or taking it as a supplement is a surefire way to balance blood sugar. That's why it's also in GOLDEN BALANCE. The liver plays a huge role in blood sugar balancing, breaking down hormones, and detoxifying your body.

Here are a few ways I love to modify my GOLDEN BALANCE:

1. **Customizing Your Drink:** The best part about GOLDEN BALANCE is its flexibility. You can tailor your drink to your liking and add the nutrients your

body needs. Whether you want to increase the fat, protein, or even fiber content, GOLDEN BALANCE can accommodate it all.

2. **Increasing Fat Content**: To make your GOLDEN BALANCE more indulgent, use coconut cream as your base. This will give your drink a creamy and delicious texture. Other options for added fats include MCT oil, ghee, or even organic butter. Each of these adds a savory note and boosts the fat content of your drink.

3. **Adding Protein:** If you want to increase the protein content of your GOLDEN BALANCE, consider adding our PRO-COLLAGEN WB powder to it. This is an easy way to supplement your protein intake and make your drink even more nourishing.

4. **Adding Other Bio-actives:** Add additional fiber with FIBER PLUS and LOVE MY GREENS to suit your medical needs.

5. **Creating a Creamy Texture:** To achieve a creamy and satisfying consistency, use a foamer to blend all ingredients. This will result in a creamy, warm "hug in a mug," as one of our clients lovingly calls it.

Remember, your GOLDEN BALANCE is more than just a drink; it's an adjustable hug in a mug that caters to your specific nutritional needs. It's also a great reminder that you can bookend your day by drinking it.

There are many ways to modify GOLDEN BALANCE and make it yours. You may even find that you just want GOLDEN BALANCE straight up, mixed in with some milk of your choice, and eat a fat bomb or a little bit of leftover dinner.

That's another great way to use medical food to balance your blood sugar all night.

I hope that through Kristen's story, you can see how crucial it is for all types of different symptoms to prevent the swings from high to low blood sugars. Mastering blood sugar balance is critical to every single one of your health symptoms. I've listed many health symptoms and diagnoses related to having a significant blood sugar swing problem throughout this lesson. I want to point out that the list of symptoms or diagnoses is by no means exhaustive. In fact, it's not hyperbole to say what I've talked about in terms of the number of symptoms related to blood sugar swings is a drop in the bucket. It's difficult for me to think of any diagnosis or symptom that doesn't have blood sugar as one of its root causes.

No matter what that symptom is, I guarantee you 100% I can link it back to your blood sugar. How do I know that? Because I've seen every single one of my client's symptoms improve and are often eliminated by blood sugar mastery.

Now, let's dive into symptoms that, to me, are tell-tale signs of blood sugar instability.

## Insomnia as a Tell-Tale Sign

Do you have trouble falling asleep? What about staying asleep? If so, you're not alone. Many people struggle with these issues. Falling asleep can become a nightmare long before you're in bed. It can start hours earlier with fear and panic, sending your cortisol levels soaring and making it impossible to fall asleep. This creates a vicious cycle that makes the fear of sleep even worse.

Even if you do manage to fall asleep, you may wake up in the middle of the night with palpitations, headaches, racing thoughts, or physical discomforts like pain or cramps, making it difficult to get back to sleep. These issues are all too common and can significantly hinder achieving restful, rejuvenating sleep.

Most people think this is just insomnia. And I'm here to tell you that this is low blood sugar 99.99% of the time. How does low blood sugar impact sleep? Firstly, most people are told not to eat before bed. This can be fine for most people, but not if you have the number one symptom associated with low blood sugar. One piece of generalized medical advice can be absolutely the wrong advice for someone who can't stay asleep, for example. Why?

Typically, a person with insomnia is someone who already tends to swing high and low blood sugar throughout the day. This swing of high to low blood sugar causes a huge cascade of problems. But frequently, people who have low blood sugar may have trouble falling asleep. Why? Their frequent episodes of low blood sugar put them into a high adrenaline state. They have tons of adrenaline in their system that was made by their adrenal glands, which are responding to low blood episodes. Recall low blood sugar means a death threat. The adrenals will make adrenaline.

Could you fall asleep if you were scared to death, high on adrenaline, your body thinks you're dying, and there's an active threat? Although people are tired and want to fall asleep, their body says, "No way. I've been under threat the whole day, and I'm in hyper-alert protection mode, ready to run and save your life at any moment." We do not recognize that when the body doesn't fall asleep, it's a reaction to frequent episodes or is in an episode of low blood sugar.

What about those nights when falling asleep isn't the problem, but staying asleep is? Here's the scenario: Your body drifts into slumber, but unstable blood sugar levels disrupt the peace, plummeting to a low in the midnight hours. Traditional Chinese Medicine dubs the window between 3-5 a.m. as 'liver time.' It's a period devoted to utilizing blood sugar and stored glycogen for hormone production and toxin breakdown.

In this quiet time, as the liver industriously works, utilizing sugar, glycogen, and fats, a stage is set for a sudden drop in blood sugar levels. This drop halts the liver's hormone production, signaling the adrenal glands (responsible for stress hormones) about the low blood sugar levels. In response, cortisol and adrenaline levels spike, diminishing the sleep-inducing hormone, melatonin.

The result? A rude awakening in the middle of the night. With escalated levels of cortisol and adrenaline and a dip in soothing hormones like melatonin, you might experience racing thoughts, hot flashes, anxiety, heart palpitations, or a sudden need to urinate – a rare occurrence for deep sleepers. This cascade of reactions, triggered by low blood sugar, converts people into light sleepers, heightens stress hormone production, and exacerbates feelings of anxiety and restlessness throughout the night.

I lived in this scenario for over a decade before unraveling the mystery. Now, armed with this insight, you, like Kristen, can promptly implement strategies to mitigate the impact of low blood sugar on your sleep, fostering a night of uninterrupted rest.

Unfortunately, the focus around insomnia tends to be sleep aids. The cure for anxiety or irritability: antidepressants. The fear of not falling or staying asleep in itself triggers worsening anxiety and fatigue. It's a vicious cycle, but it's one that's easily changeable as you read on.

## Brain Fog and ADD as Symptoms of Blood Sugar Instability

Brain fog is a real issue for men, women, children, people with attention deficit disorder (ADD), autism spectrum, sensory processing, and menopausal. It's not fake; it's real. I experienced tons of brain fog postpartum after the delivery of my child. Many I've worked with, like me, experience worsening brain fog as an adult.

In my case, I had just delivered my first child and was working my first job as a new family physician. With little sleep and a new job, I thought the brain fog was natural. Many people and doctors blamed it on being postpartum. But it didn't get better, and it continued to get worse.

I was in my late 30s. I was a highly functioning family physician and a medical director at a medical clinic, and brain fog hit me hard. To the point where I was even wondering, "Do I have ADD?" Typically, we see diagnoses in children. But more and more, we're seeing it as a diagnosis in adults. The question is, were we underdiagnosing ADD in adults? Or are we misdiagnosing adults with ADD who have blood sugar swings causing brain fog and memory problems?

Brain fog is real, and it can come in many shapes and forms, including a medical diagnosis like ADD. A medical practitioner may call distractibility ADD. But many of you reading right now have brain fog, and you weren't born with it. At some point, it came about.

How do low blood sugar episodes result in brain fog? Your brain needs a steady stream of sugar to fuel its function. High blood sugar is a brain irritant. I'd go so far as to say sugar is an excitotoxin on brain cells. Excitotoxins are molecules that overstimulate brain neuron receptors. Neuron receptors allow brain and nerve cells to communicate with each other, but when excitotoxins overstimulate them, they fire their impulses at such a rapid rate as to become exhausted or fatigued. For example, when you eat some sugar, an immediate effect may be an increase in energy or alertness followed by fatigue and poor focus. Sugar exhausts nerve and brain cells.

Take kids, for example; notice at a party full of sugar the crazy-making high level of energy they have. But they are soon followed by irritability, anger, and tears. Or these kids will crash physically at some point later in the day. Caffeine can be an excitotoxin, so you can see people who have exhaustion or withdrawals from that level of overstimulation. The effects of excitotoxins like high sugars are dose-dependent. The higher the dose, the bigger the fall. The more frequent the dose, the more frequent or chronic the fall or exhaustion. So this is not just a mechanism on how rapid, extreme blood sugar swings can cause ADD or poor focus symptoms. But clearly shines a light on how the same mechanism can cause periods of anxiety or irritability. Chronically depleted nerve cells will cause lower brain-healthy mood hormones, causing long-term depression. Brain fog is a state of brain neuron exhaustion as a result of repeated episodes of blood sugar swings.

Unfortunately, conventional medicine has no diagnostic skills to diagnose the cause of brain fog, irritability, anxiety, depression, or ADD. How many of you or your kids experience any of these symptoms and have been told your labs are normal? They are, but none of those labs are able to test for people who have big, frequent blood sugar swings. They just have clear-as-day symptoms and results that nobody recognizes the real cause of.

Kristen was able to end her anxiety and irritability within weeks. It took me years to realize my adult diagnosed ADD was because of my blood sugar swings. But once I realized it, I was able to stop my Concerta medication and be better focused without it.

Let's be clear: I'm not against medication as one tool. It's also clear some people need it. However, far fewer people would need it if they balanced their blood sugars.

Kristen's end to her anxiety and the end to my ADD and the case studies of hundreds of clients I've worked with prove without a doubt that there is an overdiagnosis and overmedication of those with ADD and mental health disorders. It speaks to the fact that brain fog is not an inevitable symptom of just giving birth or menopause.

There is a blood sugar issue that's at the root cause of it that should not be ignored. And the results from doing that are nothing short of stunning and life-changing.

## Pain is about Blood Sugar

Another symptom we're going to talk about is pain. Most people, including physicians, don't associate increased pain with blood sugar swings. Pain can come in many forms - joint or muscle pain, nerve pain (neuropathy), or even pain from an irritated nerve.

How do blood sugar swings cause pain? I'm going to bring you back to the adrenal gland that makes stress hormones. One mechanism is that low blood sugar swings cause your adrenals to perceive a death threat, and it makes cortisol and adrenaline. Elevated levels of adrenaline are known to sensitize your nerves to pain. Cortisol, the other hormone that increases during low blood sugar episodes, has been shown to produce signals of pain from peripheral nerves in the absence of an injury to that nerve.

For example, when you wake up in the middle of the night with leg pain. Or waking up with a headache in the early morning. How about episodes of nerve pain that are worse in the late afternoon? The stress hormones from cortisol and adrenaline are medically making the perception of pain worse. You're not crazy, but your blood sugar swings are, and it's making the perception of pain worse.

High blood sugar, as you recall, is an excitotoxin on the neurons or nerve cells throughout your body and in your brain. When sugars swing high, it excites and fires nerves. How many of you have neuropathy? The pain you experience is due to irritated nerves, like for those with pinched nerves in low back or neck pain. Many autoimmune diseases have the immune system attacking, firing, and damaging nerves. For example, those with lupus, Sjögren's, rheumatoid arthritis, chronic inflammatory demyelinating polyneuropathy, vasculitis, and trigeminal neuralgia all have an immune system that is attacking their nerves.

Let's go back to Kristen's story; she had two known autoimmune diseases, lupus and Sjögren's, both of which I knew were associated with chronic pain and nerve-related pain.

Having dealt with thousands of clients with autoimmune diseases, including myself, I can say with 100% accuracy that no matter what autoimmune disease one has been diagnosed with, the immune system is always attacking other targets of autoimmune attack. Think of it this way: if your immune system is mistaking one part of your body as a germ and is actively trying to kill it, how could it not also be doing this with any other target through the body? That is why anyone with any autoimmune disease with chronic pain is almost sure to have some level of attack against their nerves, causing a neuropathy related to an autoimmune attack. Seeing any diagnoses of autoimmune disease with chronic pain in Kristen directly pointed at nerve overstimulation, which is directly worsened by, you've guessed it, blood sugar swings. The point is, if you have any degree of chronic pain, don't assume it's just related to a joint or muscle problem; it's frequently associated with nerve and nerve pain. So, understanding how nerves can overfire as a result of blood sugar swings goes a long way.

Another part of Kristen's story revolves around her headaches, a pain resonating in the head or brain, regions full of nerves. The pressing question is, can fluctuations between high and low blood sugar levels act as a catalyst for headaches? Indeed, this roller coaster of blood sugar levels can exacerbate the frequency and intensity of chronic headaches, serving as a major clue in her case study.

Observe the timing of these headaches. It often unveils a huge clue. Those who frequently awaken with headaches are frequently the same individuals who are jolted awake in the night due to episodes of low blood sugar. This pattern, as Kristen's story illustrates, is a common and shared experience.

I highly recommend taking a few days of a pain or symptom journal. Notice when pain symptoms occur, and I mean any pain or discomfort. Don't dismiss headaches, numbness or tingling, or even abdominal pain.

In Kristen's case, her gut is full of nerves, and they don't move properly when she encounters blood sugar swings brought on by these fluctuations in her nervous system. Yes, her swallowing and gastroparesis were caused by blood sugar swings. This may even include abdominal pain and irritable bowel syndrome. By starting to see when these pain episodes occur, you may start to notice it immediately follows a high carbohydrate meal, or it's after a period of prolonged not eating. In our programs, we do take deep dives into food journals and symptom tracking.

A great start here is just to track the timing of your various pain symptoms and start seeing where the pattern occurs. In this way, you'll start making the connection that it is not random when pain occurs; there is a link to other root causes, including the main one, blood sugar.

# Blood Sugar Swings Trigger Mast Cell, Histamine, and Allergic Reactions

As we shift our focus to allergies and food reactions, an increasing number of individuals experience related symptoms like allergies, food sensitivities, mast cell activation disorder, and histamine intolerance. If you suffer from any of these, it's crucial to know that blood sugar levels can worsen your allergy symptoms, regardless of whether they are food-related or not. People who experience blood sugar swings often face aggravated allergy symptoms. This makes managing blood sugar levels all the more crucial for people with allergies.

This will be explored in depth in the lesson on infection and the microbiome. Suffice it to say that when blood sugar swings high, it feeds infectious organisms that make histamines. This will increase other reactions to food and environmental allergens. When the infectious organisms inside you make more histamine, then it doesn't take much more to create a reaction. Sugar feeds infection, which increases histamines.

Low blood sugar starves these organisms, which will cause a die-off cycle. As organisms like bacteria, fungus like Candida, or parasites are starved of sugar, some will die. This will release their insides, and that's allergenic, triggering histamines to rise again.

The key for this lesson is that high and low blood sugars cause the rise and fall of infectious organisms, which will cause episodes of histamine release. So, believe it or not, one of the keys to ending mast cell, histamine intolerance, and any allergic disorder is to reduce the number of times your blood sugar swings from high to low and vice versa.

I've worked with and helped turn around so many people with impossible-to-treat mast cell, histamine, or food allergy-related symptoms that I've created a whole multipart training on it along with case studies. It's part of the bonus kit included in this book!

## Postural Orthostatic Tachycardia Syndrome (POTS), Dysautonomia, Dizziness, and Vertigo are Caused by Blood Sugar Swings

You only need to read this section if you likely have POTS or dysautonomia. One of the mystery sets of symptoms that confound doctors and patients alike are those having to do with dizziness, racing heart, fainting, positional changes making things worse, blood pressure shifts going up or down, and even those with tinnitus, ringing in their ears. Frequently, the lab work is normal.

Sometimes, they're sent to specialists who do tilt table tests and other testing for further diagnosis. For those "lucky" enough to have a diagnosis, they frequently get medications that don't help, or they get no help. For example, POTS is considered by many doctors to be an untreatable chronic problem, and there's no cure.

That is not my experience. Some doctors working on underlying causes, like I do with blood sugar, hormones, and infection, have seen dramatic permanent changes for those with this and other related conditions. Here's one typical case.

*Dina is a 25-year-old marketing executive for a nonprofit. She struggled with worsening POTS symptoms, mast cell activation syndrome, and many food allergies. She also had bouts of insomnia, anxiety, and depression. This was impacting her ability to perform at her job. This also made her incredibly anxious and fearful of walking, driving, and daily outings. As a young person in her twenties, this impacted her social life as well as limiting her social and emotional connection with others. She had heavy and irregular periods and severe acne with dramatic weight loss. This made her extremely conscious about her appearance, affecting her sense of self-confidence and trust in her own abilities.*

*After two months of working with me, I was speaking with Dina, and she gasped when she realized she hadn't had a single one of her POTS-related symptoms for over a month. There was no more dizziness and difficulty with walking or driving. She was able to get up and sit down without any instability. She was bewildered when she said, "Dr.Maggie, my POTS symptoms have been gone for over a month!"*

*Not only did Dina turn around her POTS symptoms, but today, her mast cell activation and histamine intolerance reactions associated with food and smells are also gone.*

*She's now eating out, cooking, and enjoying life. And she did it by mastering her blood sugar. She shares in multiple interviews how neither she nor her specialists ever predicted that those unsolvable problems would be solved through blood sugar balance. She's working full time, excelling at her job, and in a very healthy, happy relationship. She not only feels great inside, but her skin acne has cleared up, and she's gaining healthy weight and is exercising.*

Like Kristen's story, which we talked about earlier, what are the clues to highlight about blood sugar that I saw in her original set of symptoms? Highlight her symptoms of dizziness, problems with blood pressure with positional changes, fast heart rate runs, anxiety, worsening allergy symptoms, and we later also discovered a rip-roaring gut infection. These are all related to blood sugar issues. Using her case study, I want to highlight how dizziness, positional blood pressure and heart rate changes, and vertigo with loss of balance can all be clearly triggered by blood sugar swings.

How does blood sugar swings affect blood pressure? Low blood sugar, as you recall, elicits a fight or flight response from your adrenals. The adrenals make cortisol and adrenaline. Adrenaline is known to trigger vasoconstriction, which is a contraction of the blood vessels in some areas and the dilation of others. Imagine in fight or flight; your body wants to increase blood flow to the arms and legs to run while decreasing the blood flow to normal metabolism muscles. So, fight or flight causes significant blood flow and blood pressure swings. It also activates your heart to beat faster to get ready to pump more blood.

This causes increased and sometimes irregular heart rates.

Matt, 28, suddenly fainted during a class we both attended. Alarmingly, this was the third time in just two weeks he experienced a rapid, irregular heartbeat known as atrial fibrillation. He had foregone breakfast that day and consumed two cups of coffee, which set off his fainting spell and accelerated heart rate. As I assisted Matt, I managed to stabilize his heart rate and help him regain consciousness. What stood out was that this severe blood sugar fluctuation was a central concern. Surprisingly, after his initial episodes, a holistic nutritionist advised him to adopt a vegetarian or vegan diet.

Consequently, he consumed minimal protein or fats, relying mainly on carbohydrates. While many champion these diets for their health benefits, if they are predominantly carbohydrate-based, they fail to stabilize blood sugar, leading to significant fluctuations. As previously illustrated by Dina's case, such blood sugar peaks and valleys can exacerbate cardiovascular symptoms, making them more recurrent.

Unfortunately, Matt's situation, while extreme, is not uncommon. When the root problem—blood sugar swings—isn't accurately identified, well-intentioned dietary advice can inadvertently worsen the symptoms. Adopting a healthful diet doesn't necessarily mean it's suitable for blood sugar management. Currently, Matt is under the care of a cardiologist to eliminate any potential heart-related issues, a typical step for those with rapid heart rates and fainting episodes.

Yet, mirroring Dina's experience, I anticipate many individuals with erratic heart rhythms, fainting, and blood pressure shifts often leave these consultations without any concrete answers, with stress often cited as the primary cause.

Some may even be prescribed medications for blood pressure or heart rate regulation, which could exacerbate the blood pressure shifts, dizziness, or fainting spells. For Matt, his recovery journey is ongoing, but there's already noticeable improvement. Discover more about his story in the section below.

Many cardiovascular experts firmly believe that medications are the sole solution for addressing cardiovascular concerns, including heart rate, rhythm, and blood pressure anomalies. This viewpoint is concerning, given the profound influence of blood sugar swings on overall health. Hence, achieving and maintaining stable blood sugar levels—without extreme highs or lows—is what I term "blood sugar mastery."

Dina's story is a testament to the transformative power of stable blood sugar levels. Through countless interviews, she consistently highlights the importance of maintaining her blood sugar equilibrium as the linchpin of her health transformation. Blood sugar mastery isn't just about regulation; it's about dominion. It means taking command of your blood sugar every moment of the day, ensuring it doesn't dictate the terms of your health.

Dina's journey with fluctuating blood sugar was a gradual one, undermining her well-being bit by bit. In contrast, Matt's ordeal was abrupt, presenting immediate life-threatening symptoms demanding swift intervention. Observing these two individuals at different phases in their health journeys has been enlightening. Dina, having regained her health, is now committed to sharing her insights and solutions with others. After assisting Matt during that critical episode at the conference, we've had multiple discussions. He's currently undergoing a comprehensive medical evaluation and has also been reviewing a preliminary version of this book.

The results are promising: Matt has implemented significant changes and is on the mend, with no recurrence of his previous symptoms.

## Conclusion

Kristen, Dina, and Matt's stories highlight some of the most common symptoms as a result of blood sugar swings from high to low. Many of these typical tell-tale signs of blood sugar instability were highlighted in this lesson. Review all the symptoms you highlighted in their stories. Do they mirror some of your symptoms?

The key to blood sugar mastery is to balance your plate with macronutrients of fat, protein, and fiber.

The other concept, to begin with, is how to bookend the day using breakfast and before-bed snacks or medical foods.

I've enclosed in the appendix a sample blood sugar balanced day meal plan that exemplifies the balanced plate.

I've also included a worksheet for meal planning on a blood sugar-balanced day.

If this book is your first introduction to me, you should know I'm a foodie! I love to cook, and I love food. If you're interested in seeing me cook and talk about food, there are videos on our YouTube channel as well as a companion recipe guide available.

Are you beginning to draw links between blood sugar fluctuations and various symptoms or conditions such as POTS, dysautonomia, mast cell activation syndrome, histamine intolerance, chronic pain, neuropathy, persistent headaches, gut issues, chronic fatigue, ADD, mental fogginess, and other mental health concerns? You're on the right track. Dive into our YouTube channel. There, you'll find detailed case studies showcasing individuals who, like you, have achieved truly out-of-the-box health results.

## Action Steps

1. Balance your plate with macronutrients: fat, protein, and fiber.
2. Eat carbohydrates, starchy sugar foods last in your meal.
3. Add acids like lemon or vinegar to carbohydrates or DIGEST-IT to a meal to slow the release of glucose or sugar into your bloodstream.
4. Go to the Appendix to review the balanced meal recommendations.
5. Review the meal planning worksheet to help plan meals for the day.
6. Check out my recipe book of balanced meals and snack ideas.
7. Bookend the day with breakfast within an hour of awakening and end the day with a snack before bed.
8. Make things easy with medical foods like GOLDEN BALANCE and variations of it available at www.mymdshop.com

9. Included in the Appendix is a recipe section: I've included several unique recipes to bookend your day
    - High Fat Green Smoothie
    - Protein Smoothie
    - Transform Power Breakfast: Rice, Kim Chi, Greens, and an Egg
    - Chia Seed Pudding
    - Coconut Fat Bombs

10. Check out our entire library on our YouTube channel for a full playlist of case studies and trainings around blood sugar mastery @DrMaggieYu.

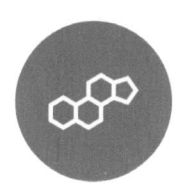

# LESSON 6:
# "IT'S JUST YOUR HORMONES..." "IT CAN'T BE YOUR HORMONES."

So, which is it?

Nearly 40% of people are prediabetic. Nearly 80% of them and their doctors are unaware of it. Worse yet, by the time they and their doctor are aware of it, the patient is blamed as if it's their fault. Somehow, in their ignorance about this, they've caused this problem. The problem with this common scenario is that diabetes is a hormone problem. It's a condition related to high blood sugar that's caused by underlying hormone imbalances, and there are often genetics involved. That's why it tends to hit certain age groups and hormonally charged times. This is also why it runs in certain families or ethnic groups. It is your hormones, and it's not your fault.

In this lesson, we're going to explore the role of times of hormonal change that turns the on and off switch on many different symptoms. You will also understand the inherent bias in our medical system, blaming everything on hormonal change while, at other times, dismissing its importance entirely.

*A female physician had her first baby at the age of 30. She had gestational diabetes, which was managed with diet. After the delivery, she developed a mastitis breast infection while breastfeeding and took antibiotics. After the antibiotics, she developed mucus diarrhea, which turned out to be a C. Difficile infection resistant to multiple rounds of antibiotics. During this time, she developed severe postpartum depression, weight gain, and insomnia.*

*While pregnant with her second child, she discovered she had insulin-dependent gestational diabetes. Postpartum, she developed intense brain fog, leading to a diagnosis of ADD, painful right shoulder and arm pain, and later diagnosed with fibromyalgia. At 35, she noticed the absence of her periods. At 36, her colleagues diagnosed her with early menopause and wrote off many of her symptoms as being not hormone-related with a single Follicle-Stimulating Hormone (FSH) test.*

*In frustration with her colleagues' dismissal of her growing list of symptoms, she learned how to test her own hormones and took it upon herself to understand how a 37-year-old woman could have early menopause and this slew of physical and mental health symptoms. This led her to discover her hormonal imbalance and her hidden Hashimoto's and autoimmune disease.*

*This story has resonated with hundreds of thousands worldwide. Since that time, she's helped diagnose and treat thousands of men and women with hidden hormonal imbalances that were the underlying root cause of many of their symptoms. This story is my story.*

Stepping into the realm of functional and natural medicine was prompted mainly by my early menopause at age 36. It wasn't just the cessation of my periods for two years; it was the accompaniment of severe fibromyalgia pain, digestive issues, anxiety, depression, irritability, and pronounced brain fog. The latter was so crippling that it undermined my performance as a medical director at a clinic.

During my personal journey, I developed a deep understanding of the crucial role hormones play in our lives. Their impact isn't limited to just reproductive functions; they significantly influence our overall quality of life and longevity. I came to realize that ovarian hormones like estrogen, progesterone, or testosterone don't solely define our hormonal spectrum. When I was diagnosed with Hashimoto's, an autoimmune disease that affects the thyroid, it underscored how shifts in thyroid hormone levels can profoundly alter mood, energy, and pain perception.

With further exploration, I understood that hormones are multifaceted actors in our body's intricate system. They aren't just about reproduction; they interconnect with other hormones throughout our endocrine system. Sex hormones interact seamlessly with our thyroid, adrenal glands, pancreas, brain, and gut, highlighting the profound links among these systems. Intriguingly, even our gut cells can produce serotonin, a hormone usually linked to the brain.

It's common for individuals to experience fluctuations in digestive symptoms, such as constipation or diarrhea, at particular times of the month. This hints at the influence of sex hormones on gut function. Regrettably, conventional medical doctors often under-address adrenal glands, mainly due to a lack of training in most adrenal-related symptoms. Adrenal fatigue, a condition that affects many and lies in a gray area between the extremes of Cushing's syndrome and Addison's disease, is frequently overlooked.

In my observation, about 99% of doctors lack training in adrenal fatigue, leaving many patients undiagnosed and untreated despite its significant impact on quality of life and longevity. The associated symptoms can be debilitating, yet they are routinely dismissed. For those interested in delving deeper into this topic, there are hundreds of videos, training, and downloadable resources from our YouTube channel **@DrMaggieYu.**

## Symptoms Associated with Hormone Imbalances

Typically, hormonal symptoms in women are associated with insomnia, hot flashes, irregular periods, heavy periods, and PMS, while in men, they are linked to erectile dysfunction. However, numerous hormone-related symptoms in women, men, and children are often overlooked and not acknowledged as hormone-related. In the bonus tool kit with this book, there is an extensive list of hormone-related symptoms that your doctor doesn't know about. Be sure to get that list.

**Insomnia,** for example, can affect anyone at any stage, not just during perimenopause. Men may also experience insomnia or sleep apnea, impacting their testosterone production and overall hormone balance. Fatigue, another common symptom, can affect people of all ages and is not solely related to getting older. Moreover, fatigue can manifest as mental or brain fog linked to hormonal imbalances.

**Pain** is another symptom many people do not realize is connected to hormonal imbalances. Hormones play a crucial role in our overall well-being, and understanding their impact can help us address various symptoms and improve our quality of life. They believe that pain can manifest in various forms, such as fibromyalgia, injuries (both old and recent), shoulder or wrist pain due to overuse, chronic regional pain syndrome (CRPS), pain associated with autoimmune conditions like rheumatoid arthritis, and more. While it's true that pain can be linked to these conditions or injuries, I want to emphasize that certain factors can trigger or exacerbate pain syndromes. In my practice and experience, I've found that women tend to experience more pain between the ages of 35 and 55.

Additionally, pain can be diurnal (meaning it occurs at specific times of the day), which people may not even realize. For example, low blood sugar can cause more pain, such as headaches, joint pain, and muscle aches in the morning. Similarly, some people may experience more pain at night.

I love the concept of "the devil you know versus the one you don't know." In the context of blood sugar, the devil you don't know is hypoglycemia, or low blood sugar, while we typically think of high blood sugar as the primary problem. Hypoglycemia is a lesser-known issue. I dive deeper into the role of hypoglycemia in the Blood Sugar Mastery lesson.

I'm bringing this up here because hormonal change can trigger blood sugar swings. So, is there a puppet master triggering blood sugar swings? Yes. The endocrine hormone production and breakdown system in your body is the underlying reason for many health symptoms that come and go throughout your life or even your day. Hormones impact many organ systems. During times of significant hormone changes, it becomes an on-and-off switch for many health problems. Let's explore this concept of hormonally vulnerable times.

# Hormonally Vulnerable Times

There are periods when we become more susceptible to hormonal shifts; I refer to them as 'hormonally vulnerable times." What are those periods?

## Puberty

*Tyler, during his late teenage years, developed joint pain and diarrhea. He was later diagnosed with Ankylosing Spondylitis and Crohn's.*

*Esther was an 18-year-old college student with POTS and had anxiety-related diarrhea. These symptoms started when she was 16 and were worse during her periods.*

Puberty is often the time when you see an onset of new symptoms. In Tyler's case, his late teens brought significant hormone shifts, and that's when he was diagnosed with two new autoimmune diseases. I have seen a considerable correlation between when hormones change and the onset of autoimmune diseases. Take a look at Esther's case above, too; it's frequently during the teen years that we see an onset of symptoms of weight changes, mental health changes, and, in her case, changes in blood pressure, dizziness, as well as gut-related symptoms like diarrhea and food allergies.

## Monthly Menstrual Cycle

*Esther was an 18-year-old college student with POTS and had anxiety-related diarrhea. These symptoms started when she was 16 and were worse during her periods.*

There are huge monthly swings in hormones in order for women to ovulate and cycle monthly. This makes women more vulnerable to big swings in their symptoms on a monthly basis. Women during certain times of the month will experience changes in their mental health, pain, headache, and bowel habits. It's no accident that many of you are more fatigued or unfocused at certain times of the month. How many, like Esther, had unexplained worsening of her POTS symptoms right before her period? The other issue is the frequency of these hormone swings in women makes them way more susceptible and at higher risk of turning on their genes for autoimmune disease.

Did you know women have a fourfold increase in the risk of autoimmune disease compared to men? Well, women have way more vulnerable times of hormonal swings, including their monthly cycle! Highlight this puppy right here.

Apparently, nobody knows why this is the case. A recent search shows that the mechanism for this autoimmune sex bias remains obscure. There's no obscurity here. It's because women have way more frequency and intensity in the times when they have hormonal shifts. It's also by no accident that they're most likely to be diagnosed with an autoimmune disease during those times, puberty, postpartum, around menopause.

## Postpartum

*Beth gave birth to twins, and six months later, she was diagnosed with polymyalgia rheumatica, causing muscle pain throughout her body, and later Graves' thyroid disease.*

When a woman is pregnant, she immediately shuts down ovarian hormone production. In its place, other hormones elevate, like the Human Chorionic Gonadotropin (HCG) hormone. During the rise of this hormone in pregnancy, women are extremely prone to diabetes (gestational diabetes, pregnancy-related diabetes). I had this during both of my pregnancies as a result of this hormone change. Beth's case study above showed how, after she delivered her twins, she developed thyroid problems with Grave's disease and pain-related autoimmune disorder with polymyalgia rheumatica.

After the birth of a baby, a woman not only delivers the baby but also the placenta.

The placenta is a hormone-making organ as well as the nutrient supply for the baby. During the delivery of the placenta, a quick, massive drop in hormones is triggered.

This drop triggers many other hormone-related conditions, such as postpartum thyroiditis (a hormone-triggered autoimmune attack on a woman who just delivered a baby. In my case). The delivery of the baby triggered hormone shifts that caused my blood sugars to swing tremendously, causing me to have fatigue, brain fog, and, worse yet, set my body up for infections. This is the reason why so many women who just gave birth experience various types of infections, like me with mastitis, a breast infection, and later a gut infection called C. difficile.

## Perimenopause

*Lucy was a 56-year-old postmenopausal woman who felt like an 86-year-old. She had severe fatigue and no libido, developed increased allergies to food, and had a new diagnosis of irritable bowel syndrome. She had a total hysterectomy at the age of 52 due to heavy bleeding and fibroids.*

*Maggie had early menopause at the age of 36. She had several episodes of postpartum depression and infection. She was later diagnosed with Hashimoto's and Mixed Connective Tissue Disease, both autoimmune diseases.*

It's been already mentioned that women are four times more likely to get autoimmune diseases than men. According to autoimmuneinstitute.org, 78% of people affected by autoimmune disease are female.[2] There is a peak in diagnosis around the late teens, followed by one around the age of 40-50. Why? Menopause is a time of big hormonal upheavals and swings. These hormone shifts are why not just autoimmune diseases but many chronic health conditions for women start right around the time when their hormones shift in this way. The average person being diagnosed with a thyroid problem is a forty to sixty-year-old woman.

---

[2] https://www.autoimmuneinstitute.org/articles/7-risk-factors-for-autoimmune-disease/

In the above case studies, take a look at Lucy's story. She had a ton of hormonal hell with heavy periods and, as a result, had a partial hysterectomy. When someone has surgery to remove a hormone-making organ, it actually causes an abrupt hormonal change. How many of you have had a hysterectomy, partial or total, only to see your health deteriorate after that? The removal of hormone-making organs makes the shift of hormones more massive, triggering the worsening and new onset of other symptoms. Notice Lucy got worsening food allergy symptoms and irritable bowel syndrome after her hysterectomy. Does this resonate with you or someone you know?

Why are perimenopausal women getting so sick? Well, they're being ignored.

They're told, "It's just your hormones; live with it." I was told, "Maggie, it's just early menopause; live with it." Countless women come to me being told they were denied testing and respectful conversations about their symptoms because they were told it's just menopause. If you knew, and now you do know, that menopause is the known trigger and vulnerable time for the onset and worsening of most, if not all, of your health-related symptoms, would you ever say it's just your hormones? I never do because I had to live through that.

Lucy was able to talk to our team and sign up to test her hormones. She reviewed science-backed video training modules. She received her results directly and reviewed those results with a hormone expert and a functional nutritionist. She was able to truly understand her underlying hormone patterns and their root causes. It turned out she was low on everything. Not just postmenopausally low, but low enough to be 86 years old. No wonder she felt like thirty years older.

She not only got her hormones balanced and her hormone symptoms relieved. Unexpectedly, she found the answers to her food allergies to end those symptoms and her irritable bowel syndrome. Now, she's taking what she's learned to help her daughter navigate through her Polycystic Ovary Syndrome (PCOS).

### Male Hormone Shifts

*Tyler, during his late teenage years, developed joint pain and diarrhea. He was later diagnosed with Ankylosing Spondylitis and Crohn's.*

*Mark was a 27-year-old musician who developed severe social anxiety and chronic brain fog and struggled with ADD.*

*Thomas gained 20+ pounds over three years in his late 40's, along with depression and joint pains.*

Men experience hormone shifts as well, though differently than women. Consider Tyler, who remained asymptomatic until his late teens when he began experiencing pain and bowel symptoms.

Unlike women, men don't experience monthly cycles. However, they do witness daily testosterone surges, especially in the mornings.

As the day wears on, many men experience a drop in testosterone, which can exacerbate certain symptoms. It isn't unusual for men like Mark or Thomas to experience heightened anxiety or depression in the evenings, coinciding with a dip in both adrenal hormones and testosterone.

Many men grapple with a condition known as obstructive sleep apnea. Genetics play a role in the structure of our palate and the soft palate in the head and neck. Due to the unique shape of a male's face and neck, men—especially those carrying extra weight—are predisposed to this condition.

When asleep, this can cause their airway to collapse, leading to interrupted breathing and reduced oxygen intake. This not only affects their sleep but also disrupts hormone production during the night.

Much of male testosterone production takes place during sleep, explaining the morning surge. If sleep is disrupted due to conditions like chronic low blood sugar or sleep apnea, testosterone production can falter. These are two leading causes of low testosterone in men. Women can experience similar issues, but since men produce about ten times more testosterone, they're more susceptible to major fluctuations, which can lead to pronounced symptoms. A testament to this is Thomas, who, after being diagnosed with severe sleep apnea, found relief in using a CPAP machine. Within three months, his testosterone levels normalized, further illustrating the intricate relationship between sleep, weight, and hormone levels. As I've touched upon previously concerning blood sugar, low blood sugar can spur the adrenal gland to release cortisol and adrenaline. This often results in night-time awakenings. A lack of oxygen due to interrupted breathing similarly halts hormone production.

Unfortunately, many men with low testosterone remain undiagnosed. A persistent bias exists against hormone testing for both genders. Symptoms like fatigue, anxiety, and even new autoimmune diagnoses don't always prompt extensive hormone tests in men. Often, men are only screened for hormone imbalances when they exhibit severe symptoms like erectile dysfunction. This, unfortunately, means many miss out on early interventions.

So, should testing for male hormones be more accessible and precise? Absolutely. However, is testosterone replacement always the solution for men with low testosterone levels? Despite the influx of clinics offering such treatments, it might not be the ideal solution for everyone, as I'll elaborate on later.

Consider Mark, a 27-year-old whose case study is presented above. His testosterone levels were shockingly low, equivalent to a 12-year-old's. He also battled severe adrenal fatigue. Mark's story underscores the fact that hormonal shifts can happen at any age. Typically, substantial hormonal changes are observed between ages 10 to 16 due to puberty. Recognizing and understanding these hormonal shifts is crucial for understanding one's overall health and potential symptoms. If overlooked, one might miss a critical piece in the puzzle of overall well-being.

Hormonal shifts aren't limited to specific life stages. There are surges during events like puberty and significant declines, such as during menopause for women or andropause (a non-medical term referring to when male hormones can drop) for men. This hormonal vulnerability is something both genders experience.

What do all these people have in common?

They all had major health shifts at hormonally vulnerable times that their physicians missed.

The prevailing question remains: why aren't more men and women having their hormones evaluated during these times when they have the most health-related symptoms? There are many obstacles.

## Obstacles to Hormone Balance

**Lack of training & understanding** by practitioners is rampant. Regulating hormonal balance presents numerous hurdles, the most significant of which is the lack of understanding about the existence and significance of a hormonal timeline. This is unknown to the average person, and many practitioners often lack training in this critical aspect of health. Consequently, it's common to see women in their 40s struggle to find adequate healthcare due to symptoms that medical professionals cannot readily explain.

Reflecting on my career as a physician, one of my most profound realizations - and indeed, a source of significant professional regret - was the failure to connect these health issues with hormonal imbalances. I recall the many instances of seeing women in their 40s, exhausted and searching for answers. At the same time, my colleagues and I struggled to understand why they were feeling so tired when their lab results appeared normal.

Without a clear understanding of the hormonal implications, our go-to solutions were typically antidepressants, birth control pills if menstrual irregularities were reported, and therapy. However, these were rarely adequate solutions, mainly because they failed to address the underlying hormonal issues.

The fact is, these women in their 40s were experiencing a time of dramatic hormonal shift. Their hormones were dropping and changing, triggering not just fatigue but insomnia, anxiety, depression, pain, the onset of other diseases, and even cardiovascular disease. There's a reason why cardiovascular diseases like high cholesterol and high blood pressure often develop during this period. Yet, these issues are often treated as separate problems, and patients are told they'll need medications for life. The truth is that cardiovascular disease is onset around this time because of significant hormonal shifts.

The obstacle is that doctors need to gain training on the awareness that these aren't just diseases of aging; they are diseases and symptoms that are triggered to start or get worse related to times of hormonal change. We need to be looking at these vulnerable times in men, women, and children as a serious risk factor and an early warning signal of serious medical changes.

**Testing for hormones can be problematic.** There are three main ways to test for hormones: blood, saliva, and urine. Each type of testing has its advantages and disadvantages. Each type of testing requires unique training of the practitioners, and they need experience in the results themselves from performing many tests with many different types of patients to truly understand the underlying patterns of hormone imbalance. The three different testing types are not interchangeable. For example, if you're working with a doctor who uses blood work, saliva, or urine testing, they may not be testing the same form of the hormone. Many practitioners don't realize this and, therefore, can't make heads or tails out of seemingly conflicting results. In reality, they're not even testing the same things.

Take, for example, two companies are testing hormones in different ways. They both list that they are checking estrogen levels. One test is testing for the total amount of estrogen, whereas the other company is testing for free (active) hormones. They can be very different depending on the individual. As if that's not confusing enough, many medical providers don't know this. They will dismiss other providers or other test results, not understanding that the tests are not testing for the same thing.

Another issue is that blood work for hormones may be fine for testing sex hormones like progesterone, estrogen, or testosterone, but they are not great for testing adrenal hormones. Adrenal hormones need to be tested for the trend and pattern throughout the day, requiring multiple samples to be collected.

There is a lot to learn about each type of testing. Not one type of testing is necessarily better than others; they all have their pros and cons. The important thing is that you and your provider are educated in detail on the type of testing being used so that you get tested at the right time, using the test they have the most experience with, and for them to do this on thousands of individuals so that they understand how to understand the results accurately.

Unfortunately, doctors do not get this training; therefore, they and their patients are confused. So, doctors often resist ordering hormones because of their own ignorance. Later in this lesson, I'll go into what test you should order that's easiest to understand and accurate.

**Doctors don't train or offer something insurance doesn't pay for.** Many people don't realize that much of what is offered to you is directed by what insurance is willing to pay for. For example, the testing that your doctor is willing to offer you for your condition is dictated by which test is cheap, which one the insurance will cover, and which one will cause the least amount of paperwork to defend or justify.

As doctors, most of our day isn't seeing you. Most of our day is dealing with administrative work as a result of seeing you. The encounter is fifteen minutes long. More time is spent documenting in your chart for record keeping and preventing lawsuits. The most amount of time is spent billing your insurance, getting the bills rejected, and having our staff come to us asking us to fill out numerous forms to justify the payment of the labs or prescriptions. There is more staff dedicated to administration and billing than there is in direct patient care. All of these people need the doctor's time.

So, when a test costs more money than a usual blood test, it's a problem on many levels.

Firstly, doctors are rated by how much each of their patients costs in terms of the dollar amount of labs, the cost of prescriptions, and the cost of the radiological studies (x-rays, CT Scans, and MRIs) they order. Yes, each month at each of the organizations I've worked for, we received reports ranking us in relation to our colleagues. It was quick to see who's an outlier, which in a medical practice is not a good thing.

Hormone blood tests are expensive compared to other labs. Therefore, if I ordered it just once a day for one of my patients, my average cost of labs per patient would go up astronomically compared to my colleagues. Just like a restaurant would notice a server not pushing a special, organizations in healthcare and insurance companies are quick to report and reprimand doctors for being an outlier.

Added to this, patients get mad at the physician when some lab test isn't covered as they expected. A great example is that when I order a vitamin D test, which I require for every patient I care for, I tell the patient right up front, I don't know if your insurance will cover it, and even if they do, it's expensive, and you may be responsible for anywhere from $50-200 or more for this test. Here's why I need it: do you want it knowing you likely will have a bill you're not going to like? Then, I spend five minutes documenting this fact before ordering. Even then, my staff would routinely tell me about having a patient complain to them but not to me about the bill and refuse to pay. Why would I, as the physician or any of my colleagues, order an expensive hormone blood test knowing the hell I have to document and the hell my billing staff may have to deal with later? Not to add insult to injury, but after a few months of focusing on patient hormones, I'll hear from my physician medical director or the insurance company about how I'm an outlier costing the organization or the insurance company more money.

So, it's no wonder there's a tendency for physicians not to order hormone testing or any testing that isn't on the short list of the cheap 100.

As a patient, if you want your hormones tested, my advice is for you to read further on how to order and pay for your own testing. The other option is to make sure when you ask for testing to ensure the physician that you're aware that there likely is an additional out-of-pocket charge that you're more than ready to pay for. This can help overcome many layers of resistance.

**The bias against adrenal fatigue not being considered an actual medical diagnosis or problem.**
Testing adrenal fatigue solely through blood work poses challenges in capturing the daily fluctuations. On the other hand, multiple urine or saliva samples collected at different times of the day can provide more comprehensive insight into adrenal function. Relying solely on blood tests is an inadequate approach to diagnosing adrenal fatigue, which explains why many doctors are skeptical about its existence. They lack familiarity with saliva or urine testing, which offers a more practical and accurate method. Limitations are evident when hormones are assessed using a specific method, particularly blood work. Moreover, there's a lack of physician training in recognizing patterns rather than solely focusing on absolute lab values.

The adrenals serve as an excellent example to illustrate this point. Evaluating a person's adrenal function based on a single blood test for cortisol levels is insufficient and can lead to misleading conclusions. Adrenal fatigue cannot be diagnosed solely based on a one-time spot cortisol test.

Why? Because understanding hormones requires recognizing their patterns. In the case of the adrenals, there is a distinct pattern: cortisol should peak in the morning and gradually decrease as the day progresses. Variations in this pattern can indicate different stages of adrenal fatigue, underlying causes, and potential solutions.

Adrenal function is not simply a matter of being high or low; it encompasses patterns that convey a story. I could devote an entire book to this topic. In our programs, we extensively cover the intricacies of adrenal fatigue. Adrenals serve as a prime example to emphasize the significance of patterns when assessing hormones. If the testing method is inadequate, incorrect, timed inaccurately, or infrequent throughout the day, it can lead to erroneous conclusions regarding hormone levels.

Adrenal fatigue, what the pattern or phase is, gives incredible clues as to the underlying causes of many different types of diagnosis or symptoms. Take, for example, a patient with POTS. There absolutely is a typical pattern that shows up on the adrenal cortisol measurements that will point to a root cause. In the **Blood Sugar Mastery**, one of the leading causes of POTS with blood pressure and heart rate fluctuations is the effect of blood sugar on the adrenal hormones. No other physician or teacher has made this association, and it's honestly a pattern I love to teach in our programs. It's critical not to miss how the particular way these cortisol levels rise and fall isolates blood sugar swings as the main cause of these symptoms for those with dizziness, heart rate changes, and positional change-related fainting spells. I've done several result reviews on my YouTube channel, reviewing a few of these different patterns.

Many hormone specialists and doctors have experienced our programs, often commenting on the depth and nuances we offer regarding sex hormones and adrenal hormone patterns. Fellow physicians frequently ask why I delve so deeply into teaching about hormones at such an expert level. My response? An innate curiosity propelled me to master this subject. Repeatedly teaching this material thousands of times over the years has reinforced one thing: those truly ready to understand will seek out the knowledge. It's essential for everyone to realize the immense power of their hormone data. Recognizing and balancing these hormones can profoundly impact one's health.

**Hormone patterns matter more than the individual lab result.** Diving into sex hormones, we find that their patterns are even more significant than their absolute values. Patterns mean the relationships between different hormones and how they interact. Like examining a wall for its overall pattern rather than focusing on individual bricks, studying the patterns of hormones can provide more insightful information.

Take, for instance, a pattern known as estrogen dominance. This refers to a situation where estrogen is dominant relative to progesterone. It's a common misunderstanding that estrogen dominance means high estrogen levels. In this context, ' dominance' is about the ratio or relationship between estrogen and progesterone.

So, could you have low levels of both estrogen and progesterone but still exhibit estrogen dominance? Absolutely. Because it's the relative dominance of estrogen over progesterone that matters here, not the absolute levels of each hormone. Understanding this nuanced concept is key to better managing hormonal imbalances.

Unfortunately, this concept is not being taught to doctors, and thus, the general public doesn't know about it either. There is a complete lack of training for doctors to understand that estrogen dominance exists as a pattern. Yet, it is the number one trigger of many health problems for men, women, and teenagers. Our doctors don't know how to identify, test for, or understand the relationship between estrogen and progesterone. They also don't understand that estrogen dominance can occur even with low hormone levels.

Understanding and teaching the steps in hormone metabolism, how hormones are made, what they break down into, and the enzymes involved in each step is crucial. Understanding this makes it easier to identify why specific hormone patterns are the way they are and how to fix the problem. In this example, I recall Gina, who was postmenopausal and denied hormone testing because she had not menstruated for ten years. She was told she no longer needed to have her hormones tested because she hadn't had periods; of course, her hormones would be low, so why bother? And, of course, none of her rheumatoid arthritis or Hashimoto's thyroid issues had anything to do with her sex hormones. Of course, it wasn't her hormones. I tested her hormones, and they were abysmal for her age group.

Not only that, even though all her hormones were low, her estrogen was still high compared to her progesterone, so she was severely estrogen-dominant. This explained her severe hot flashes and insomnia and why she was waking up all night in pain and having gained fifteen pounds. Once her hormones were balanced so that she was no longer low on everything and estrogen-dominant, she slept through the night, and her pain level was halved. That's the power of understanding patterns and what it means to balance hormones.

**Hormone replacement does not equal hormone balance.** A major stumbling block on the path to hormone balance is the commercialization of hormone replacement therapy (HRT). Many practitioners, including functional naturopaths and doctors, position themselves as hormone experts while they profit significantly from selling hormone pellets. Individuals must comprehend that utilizing HRT in any form—pellets, orally, or patches—does not lead to hormone balance, a principle equally applicable to birth control pills. Such therapies often require doses that suppress your natural hormones, replacing imbalanced hormones with an excessive quantity, not promoting natural hormone balance.

One of the significant problems with HRT causing imbalances is the widespread lack of accurate hormone testing. This issue means doctors often fail to identify which hormones are in excess and which are deficient. Consequently, I've seen individuals with estrogen dominance being prescribed more estrogen, which should be avoided. Similarly, individuals with PCOS and estrogen dominance often have excessively high testosterone and estrogen levels and are wrongly prescribed testosterone or estrogen therapy. This happens all the time and is our "standard of care." There's no training or requirement to retest someone once they're on hormones, and there are no guidelines as to what a balanced profile should be once someone is on hormones. Many people have come to me, having been retested and told they were doing great, but they weren't. Or, they've never had a retest after being prescribed some hefty doses of hormones. Marianne had testosterone five times the amount of a woman her age. No wonder she was irritable and had acne. Yet, she was never retested.

The compensation structure for doctors also contributes to the problem. In a system where the volume of patients seen pays primary care physicians, medical solutions become constrained by what's covered by insurance. In this environment, you're likely to be prescribed medication as the primary solution—it's efficient for physicians aiming to see as many patients as possible. This model can also lead to over-prescription of hormones, worsening imbalances.

On the other hand, a cash-paying patient may choose a doctor advertising themselves as a hormone specialist. However, these practitioners often specialize in lucrative treatments like pellet therapy, not necessarily holistic hormone balance. These doctors are incentivized to recommend therapies like hormone pellet treatments over comprehensive testing or lifestyle changes because the former yields more profit. In my experience, hormone pellets are the worst option for helping anyone achieve the balance of their sex hormones. That's because they cause really high levels of hormones to circulate long-term. If it's that high, it can't easily be undone for months and months and even up to six months. Most of the advertisements you see in airline magazines and online for hormone clinics are pellet mills without any time or motivation to balance your hormones to support better health.

So, the takeaway message is two-fold: Firstly, hormone replacement therapy does not guarantee hormonal balance and can often exacerbate imbalances. Secondly, the choice of practitioner matters: ensure they understand hormone testing, timing, and underlying patterns. Most importantly, remember that most individuals do not need prescription hormones; if required, high doses are typically unnecessary and could worsen health symptoms over time. If you are in need of hormone therapy, there are low-dose options available rather than pellets or oral tablets. When receiving hormones, make sure to retest within the first three months to ensure that the dose and the balance are correct.

# How To Get Started Balancing My Hormones?

**Find a practitioner** who understands hormone balancing and patterns. Despite popular belief, only a few gynecologists and endocrinologists are experts in hormone balancing; in fact, most lack any training and will actively dismiss you. I would ideally love a specialty named functional endocrinology; however, I've only ever seen one of those providers. Unfortunately, it is precisely going to gynecologists and endocrinologists that people get the worst or no care of their hormones. You will have better prospects looking to naturopathic and functional medicine medical doctors. Some of these providers have undergone additional training to test for and balance hormones. How do you know? Visit the Institute for Functional Medicine website with their provider locator.

Check out the certifications and the website of the providers to help. I've created a few questions to help you screen the providers:

- Do you test hormones? If so, how? Blood, saliva, urine?
- Do you use hormone results to determine if someone needs hormone therapy?
- What are some of the patterns you're looking for while testing hormones?
- Have you heard about estrogen dominance or polycystic ovarian syndrome?
- Do you think postmenopausal women should have their hormones tested? If not, why not?

- Are you familiar with supplementation and lifestyle changes to balance hormones?
- Do you do hormone pellet therapy at your clinic? (If so, be very careful of the limited options of treatments they'll provide you.)
- Do you provide patient education to help me better understand my results?

If, even after going through the resources and asking the questions, you don't find the right practitioners? This is why I created MY Hormone MasterClass, where people can work with me to test and balance their hormones.

**Test your hormones accurately.** I've discussed how blood testing is insufficient and inaccurate for evaluating hormones and adrenals. I recommend doing saliva hormone testing multiple times throughout the day. If you're working with a good practitioner, they should be providing the testing. If not, empower yourself; you can order your own.

Getting the proper test ordered and knowing the right time to test it is already half the battle won. I prefer saliva testing over blood due to the better accuracy of the measurements of active hormones, and it's a great way for home collection with multiple samples throughout the day to demonstrate patterns. I do not typically recommend urine testing as the reports are far more difficult to understand, and I often see many providers misinterpret the results.

In the action items, you can learn more about how to order your own saliva hormone test kit and how to work with us directly on balancing your hormones.

**Embrace cruciferous vegetables!** They contain active compounds that aid in hormone breakdown and detoxification through the liver. In addition, these vegetables are rich in fiber, a prebiotic that nourishes the good bacteria in your gut, thus promoting overall health and influencing hormone balance. Fermentation, the final step in digestion, occurs in the large intestine, where hormones are further broken down to be eliminated. Daily bowel movements are crucial for maintaining hormonal balance. Consuming at least six cups of mostly cruciferous vegetables daily is one way to support this process. I've created and cooked several cruciferous vegetable training videos on our Youtube channel if you want to check out my hormone-balancing slaw cooking demonstration **@DrMaggieYu.**

If you have my companion recipe book, there are many recipes in the vegetable and sides section with power-packed cruciferous vegetables, and they're foodie-approved recipes. See the appendix for a sampling of a few of the recipes from the book.

**Biohack your hormones with supplementation.** Are there supplements or ingredients that are good for anyone with hormone imbalance? The answer is yes. I've created a hormone starter kit that includes supplementation and medical foods that are great for men, women, and teenagers to use.

LOVHER is great for anyone. It contains ingredients such as glucoraphanin from broccoli extract to help decrease the buildup of excessive or harmful estrogens and testosterone breakdown products. Calcium D-Glucarate helps the beneficial bacteria in the large intestine break down hormones further down the gut. Green tea extract is fantastic for testosterone and blood sugar balance. These ingredients are helpful in every type of hormone imbalance. Taking two a day is a great start.

High-quality omega-3 like PRO-OMEGA 1000 helps in the creation of hormones: the quality matters, and the quantity matters. Taking 3000mg of high-quality omega-3s is critical for many hormone balances and symptoms relating to insomnia, brain fog, and anxiety.

Blood sugar and hormone balance are tied hand in hand, so using BALANCHER two in the morning is helpful in starting the day out right to facilitate the creation and balancing of hormones.

I've had hundreds of people tell us that by watching our free training on YouTube, downloading our protocols, and starting proper food and supplementation, their symptoms have all but resolved quickly. I firmly believe that proper supplementation is a great tool to have on board. I've created a free mini course called Hormone Certainty in the bonus tool kit that contains several trainings, a symptom checklist, and a tool to map your hormonal timeline.

**Learn how to balance your hormones working with us.** Brianna was a new mom with a six-month-old baby who had gained 25 pounds since delivering her baby. She was told since she stopped breastfeeding only three months prior that, she couldn't test her hormones. Her thyroid labs and dosing fluctuated wildly. She felt fatigued and anxious, and she suffered from severe constipation. She enrolled in MY Hormone MasterClass, received her saliva hormone test kit, and knew exactly the right time to test her hormones. She reviewed the video training on her own time. After receiving the results, she did a one-week review session with me and our team, including our functional nutritionist.

While reviewing her results in the review sessions, I was able to show her how she was suffering from severe PCOS. A condition she never knew she had. All the hormones she was making were turning into too much testosterone. Additionally, her adrenal patterns clearly show that she was having blood sugar swings throughout most of the early part of her day, contributing to afternoon energy and mood crashes. The hormone patterns also demonstrated a condition called fatty liver. Yes, hormone results can actually expose other underlying problems!

On her hormone retest and review session with me three months later, Brianna's liver and her hormones on the last retest were completely back to the normal range. Her fluctuating thyroid lab levels have stabilized, and she's finally feeling confident she's on the right dose.

She shared recently that she had lost 20 pounds already, and her fatigue and brain fog were gone. She was able to sleep and get back to work, where she recently received a promotion to be the head of the marketing team at her office. She had a great deal of anxiety since the birth of her child, today all of that is gone. She and her husband are waiting on the stability of these hormones for another three months before planning to get pregnant again. This time, unlike other times, the chances of another miscarriage are going to be much lower. Why? Balanced hormones mean it is easier to get pregnant and less risk of a miscarriage. Balanced hormones don't just have an immediate impact on us; they impact our fertility, pregnancy, and postpartum health.

Her case study shows how many of her symptoms and miscarriages were connected. It also demonstrates how proper testing, education, and direct medical guidance can bring dramatic change to many areas of health. Her case also shows how balancing her hormones impacted other hormone-making organs like her thyroid. Her gut health with her blood sugar and liver problems caused some of her problems with excessively high testosterone. Her solutions were lifestyle, supplementation, and proper retesting to provide new data to plan any changes and to optimally time her next conception.

## Action Steps

1. Download the bonus tool kit, which includes Certainty in Hormones, a hormone symptom checklist, and supplement recommendations and protocols. Collect your bonus tool kit and resources at www.8OutoftheBox.com/Bonus-Health
2. Reflect on your hormone timeline, and watch my hormone story on YouTube @DrMaggieYu.
3. Find a practitioner with the guided questions provided in this lesson.
4. Work with me to test, learn, and balance your hormones in MY Hormone MasterClass at www.MYHormoneMasterclass.com
5. Test your hormones with our Hormone and Saliva test kits available at https://mymdshop.com/products/hormones-and-adrenal-saliva-kit
6. Eat 6 cups of cruciferous vegetables a day; a great example is in the appendix of our recipe for Cabbage Slaw.
7. Learn about supplementation in the numerous pieces of training on our MYMD Bio-Therapeutics Youtube channel @mymdshop

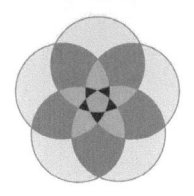

# LESSON 7:
## CREATING EXPERIENCES FOR YOUR HEALTH TRANSFORMATION

*Maryanne is a mother of three who worked for a large food distributor. She and her family had recently moved to Miami for her new job. Within six months of working in that position, one day, she got dizzy and, a few weeks later, didn't even have the energy to get out of bed. Over the next three years, she was diagnosed with multiple autoimmune diseases, infections, and mystery symptoms, including Sjögren's, Raynaud's, Epstein Barr Viral Syndrome, irritable bowel syndrome, autonomic dysfunction to the point of being bedridden by the age of 41.*

*Both she and her husband, Dan, were well-educated, highly productive individuals who thought they had health care. What they ended up realizing was that she was participating in sick care. Where doctors, many of them, and programs became documentarians of her sickness. She became another one of the patients passively receiving care from specialists and natural doctors. They often found themselves waiting for the next great test, the next great medication, and the next great naturopathic physician with the right sick diagnosis that'd transform her from bedridden back to her normal, happy, relaxed, vibrant self.*

*Instead, it was the nightmare where she became obsessed with being fearful of everything and everyone. Fear dominated and ruled her. They knew that passively receiving more sick care and researching more and more information without experiences to counter her sickness and her thoughts did not work.*

*Her husband supported her so much in helping her make the decisions that the priority in their lives is about experiences. They had never thought about putting their time and effort into an immersive experience for Maryanne until they found our program. The ritual of sick care with sick doctors, whether they're in white or green coats, didn't change her outcomes. They also realized, after speaking with us, that the system of different experiences required for her to go from being bedridden for years to being active and going places for more and more experiences to continue her life transformation.*

*I am happy to report that Maryanne is now, three years later, currently on a cruise with her family. She's shifted from fear and "I can't" to meeting with me and other alumni for a meet-up experience I recently did in Orlando. Yes, we had fun and connected until 1 a.m. Her husband shared with me that none of this health and life transformation would've happened had they not realized and made the decision to seek out experiences that would teach, motivate, and support them in taking action.*

One of the profound challenges with our healthcare perspective is that many of us adopt a reactive stance. We're conditioned to be passive beneficiaries of "sick care" only when symptoms strike. It's as if we're programmed to sit and wait for health issues to arise and then scramble for an instant, quick fix.

When you sift through most health information, the emphasis is on treatment rather than prevention. It's a cycle of waiting: waiting for the right guidance, the scheduled doctor's appointment, the relevant tests, and then the prescribed medication. Even in natural medicine, the shift is subtle.

Instead of conventional drugs, the prescription becomes a more holistic alternative, often termed "the green solution." Yet, whether it's traditional medicine or holistic remedies, the core idea remains a passive stance awaiting an inevitable outcome.

My vision deviates from this conventional blueprint. I'm not here to regurgitate textbook information or to parrot memorized solutions. While foundational knowledge is vital, it isn't the catalyst for profound transformation. So, what ignites change? Experiences!

## Experiences, Specifically Experiential Learning

Experiential learning is more than a buzzword. This approach isn't confined to the classroom; it's, in fact, the opposite. Experiential learning is like the rock star of learning methods. It's not about just hearing or reading stuff; it's about diving in and doing things for yourself. It's all about hands-on experiences and applying what you know to real-life situations. It extends to various aspects of our lives, from personal development to professional growth. In redefining what health care is versus sick care. One of the most essential systems to do that is to understand how important it is for you to have healthcare experiences that teach you the tools, thinking patterns, strategies, and tactics you need to live in wellness. You need to feel great now and to prevent any sickness in the future. The most powerful and only way to achieve this is through experiences that teach you how to do this.

Historically, both patients and doctors have been ensnared in the confines of the "sick care" narrative. To redefine and champion a proactive approach to health, we need to understand the art of curating and participating in transformative health experiences. That was the inception of "Transform," a platform dedicated to forging your health metamorphosis.

## The Pillars of Experiences for Transformation

In our journey to understand the core tenets of experiential learning, we uncover the five pillars that underpin this transformative process. These pillars—engagement, reflection, critical thinking, application, and transfer—form the framework that propels us from passive recipients of information to active participants in our own development.

Here's an example of one of our programs and how each layer creates different types of experiential learning:

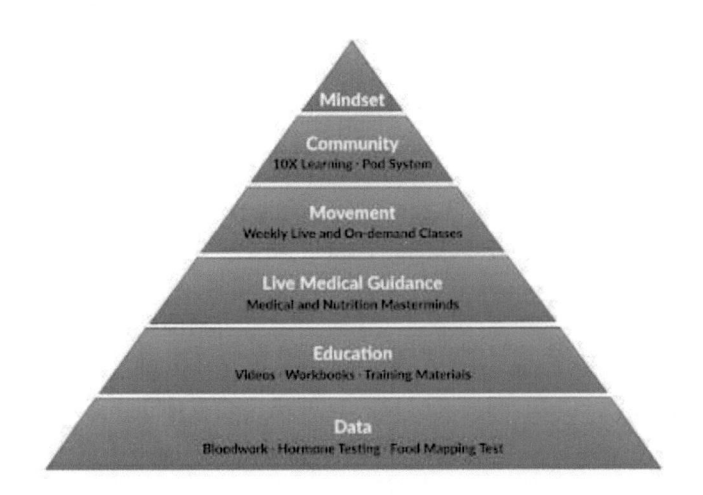

**Mindset**

**Community**
10X Learning · Pod System

**Movement**
Weekly Live and On-demand Classes

**Live Medical Guidance**
Medical and Nutrition Masterminds

**Education**
Videos · Workbooks · Training Materials

**Data**
Bloodwork · Hormone Testing · Food Mapping Test

# From Knowledge to Transformation

Transformation in health is more than just gathering facts; it embodies a fundamental shift in our mindset, emotions, and actions. Experiential learning thrusts us into the midst of real-life scenarios, sparking our curiosity and empowering us to unearth knowledge in a deeply personal way. The foundational step in this process is obtaining your health data. Personalized healthcare becomes tangible and meaningful only when grounded in your unique data—removing the realm of conjecture and placing you in the driver's seat of your own health journey.

Engaging directly with your data—feeling its weight, visualizing its patterns, and understanding its nuances—is an experience unparalleled in its richness. Our programs are unique in offering participants this hands-on opportunity. We offer detailed access and guidance on the specific labs and metrics that will best inform and enhance your learning.

Navigating the vast expanse of health data can be daunting, akin to trekking through an uncharted forest.

But we're here to be your compass, pointing out which data landmarks deserve your attention amidst the sea of information. Some data points weave intricate tales, exposing links that may have previously eluded you. Together, let's uncover these pivotal revelations.

For instance, with just four specific laboratory blood tests, we collaborated with a client and her support group to pinpoint the root causes behind her persistent dizziness, chronic fatigue, and intense food allergies that lingered for over six years. The question then arises: What is the value of accurate blood tests, precise guidance, and targeted action in unveiling mysteries that have stumped others for so long? Such is the transformative power of truly experiencing data.

## The Role of Flipped Virtual Learning

In traditional settings, many envision education as being bound within the four walls of a classroom. However, our unique approach turns this idea on its head. With our system, you engage in didactic learning at your leisure, virtually, moving through training modules at a pace that suits you. The twist? Once you've grasped the basics, you then join our live Mastermind sessions, where the real magic happens. Here, the focus shifts to implementation and personalization, ensuring you truly embody what you've learned. It's a hands-on experience, and it's all live.

You see, in typical school or online learning setups, students absorb knowledge in class and then retreat to their homes to grapple with homework and apply what they've learned. However, this model is ill-suited for health care. That's precisely why we've chosen to flip the script. There's a profound difference between rote memorization and lived experience. When you've personally navigated a situation or witnessed another do so, it imprints deeply.

You recall the emotional nuances, the narrative arc, and the lessons gleaned. This kind of experiential learning is potent and enduring. Our clients can attest to this; they never resort to mere memorization. Instead, they draw from their reservoir of personal experiences and the powerful stories of others, effectively "playing" with the concepts at hand. This leads to a depth of understanding that's both intimate and impactful.

## The Role of Physical Movement

One of the keys to creating learning experiences is that you have to pair the learning with a change in thought, word, and movement. We provide movement opportunities that are neurologically rewiring you for activity, excitement, fun, and calm. None of these states or emotions has been tied to your sick care before because this is what health care is about. It's active.

It is exciting to see and feel those big aha's. And can it be fun, exciting, and at other times calming? How would that feel in relation to your health? Fantastic. Well, there are somatic touch and movement activities that you do on a daily basis that are doable and fast tracks you to health faster and deeper! Small movements throughout your learning experiences will rewire your body and your brain! The movement and the physical experiences solidify and propel the health and mind transformation!

## The Role of Connection

Connection is not just an interaction; it's an experience, a sentiment deeply embedded in our very nature. The more attuned we are to ourselves, the more energy we derive from bonding with others. While solo endeavors have their value, shared experiences amplify our sensations tenfold. A multitude of studies affirm that collaborative activities significantly enhance individual effort and output. This is why our healing journey integrates communal experiences, teaching participants lifelong bonding skills.

My own healing chronicle underscores the impact of connection. During the toughest times, feelings of loneliness prevailed. Conversely, times of rapid healing were intertwined with shared experiences. Not only did I witness transformative effects in my life, but I also observed it in others around me.

Take Maryanne and Dan, for instance. Maryanne admitted that initially, the sheer thought of revealing her vulnerabilities – whether it was showing her face or admitting she was tucked into bed – petrified her. Dan discerned that her phobia of connecting was the very chain exacerbating her sickness. Despite these barriers, what stood out about Maryanne was her receptiveness. A burning commitment to her well-being and that of her family fueled her journey. Over the years, she recognized that her old strategies were not only ineffective but also compounded her symptoms.

In moments of vulnerability, it's the strings of connection that anchor us. Reaching out, seeking assistance, building bridges with others—these are the pillars of our healing. Our programs are intentionally designed around this ethos. We immerse participants in shared experiences, laying the foundation for profound, lasting healing. The bonds we nurture are the bedrock of our collective transformation.

*"Vulnerability is the birthplace of love, belonging, joy, courage, empathy, and creativity. It is the source of hope, empathy, accountability, and authenticity. If we want greater clarity in our purpose or deeper and more meaningful spiritual lives, vulnerability is the path."*

-Brené Brown

# The Role of Mastering Your Mind

At the pinnacle of experiences that create transformation is the need to grow your mind. No transformation anywhere in your life can happen without transformation in your mind first. That's why tools, steps, implementation, and the practice of working that muscle of growing and expanding your mind are integral to all our experiences. It's a tall order; no sick care doctor or program is going to do that.

People and programs that don't engage in mind growth are not capable of growing your mind. We can't help someone with something we are not doing ourselves. We can't deliver on a promise if it's not a core value we live, eat, breathe, or get healthy with. So, growth is my highest core value, and the only way to grow is to start with your mind first. Look who's got growth as their core value; look who is creating those experiences in you. The only way to grow through the discomfort that's in our mind is by creating human experiences that are unforgettable in how they make us feel.

The lesson **From Mindset to Mind Growth** is dedicated to helping you to better understand what mind growth is and how those experiences are essential to get health and life transformation.

# Why You Hold the Key to Navigating Your Own Data-Driven Approach

Dealing with complex medical diagnoses and symptoms can be an overwhelming journey, often requiring a multidisciplinary approach to healthcare. Traditional medical doctors may struggle to navigate holistic methods, while some holistic practitioners may not fully understand conventional medicine. Even when working with functional medicine providers, patients may find that no single expert possesses the breadth of knowledge required to address all aspects of their health. Most turn to the internet. That's become an isolating experience where people still don't get an outcome.

I've detailed the understanding and layers of experiential learning. Here's the critical piece: those experiences don't currently exist with any medical provider, healthcare system, or program. I had to create it. It is a unique signature system designed for everyone who wants to become the active driver of their health care.

In the complex health domain, a company that offers learning experiences aimed at genuine health transformations becomes a crucial ally. This positions individuals at the helm of their own health journey.

We set the stage for these transformative moments, but you need to recognize your goals, discern your needs, and put these experiences at the forefront. Breaking the cycle of bouncing between healthcare providers rests in your hands.

Many are left wandering, uncertain of their true needs, until they encounter an experience that illuminates both the "why" and the "how." It's my hope that this book kindles a deep-seated drive in you, pushing you toward pivotal experiences that champion personal growth.

Health care is not a one-size-fits-all—health care: your health care is, in fact, highly personalized. Complex medical conditions often involve many factors, including physical, emotional, and lifestyle elements. While traditional medicine plays a crucial role in diagnosis and treatment, it does not embrace holistic approaches that consider the interconnectedness of these factors. This book highlights how using a scientific approach with natural medicine and combining that with a conventional medicine approach is transformative and necessary for difficult-to-treat symptoms.

Better yet, how about taking a scientific approach to conventional medical care and naturopathic medicine and integrating them together to create powerful experiences that push the body, mind, and spirit of each individual to grow. I've discussed the metaphor of a chrysalis.

We create the container for which you can step into experiences that will create the transformation in you. Once you understand the value of this container for experiences in true transformation, it's up to you to decide to step into a fast track to human transformation.

## Conclusion

True "health" care transcends mere treatment; it empowers individuals to be the architects of their own well-being. Throughout this chapter, we've illuminated the essence of experiential learning, encouraging everyone to take a proactive role in their health journey. It's not just about obtaining knowledge but actively immersing oneself in experiences that cater to various facets of one's health.

From understanding data's significance and appreciating the power of education to valuing live implementation, the emphasis has been on a holistic approach. We've also underscored the importance of community and nurturing one's mind and spirit. Remember Maryanne's story? Her transformation was a testament to the importance of connection and shared experiences in the path to wellness.

In embracing such a diverse range of experiences, we tap into our inherent strength, charting a path of genuine health transformation. As you move forward, I invite you to explore and immerse yourself in these dynamic experiences we've discussed. The journey to true health awaits, and you're in the driver's seat.

## Action Steps

1. Want to learn more about what "health" care experiences truly are?
   Fast-track this by scheduling a chat with one of our team members at
   www.drmaggieyu.com/apply-bk

2. Do you want to see other people's experiences as they transform? What experiences were the game changers for them? How does it feel to have connected learning and healing? Hop over to our YouTube channel to watch our case studies and group interviews.

3. Want to learn more about the science behind what we do and the system that we deliver in a presentation that's about 30 minutes? Watch this training https://go.drmaggieyu.com/start-now-bk

4. Journal on these prompts. Based on these experiences of personalized data, virtual education, live coaching & implementation, movement, community, and mind growth work, what's missing in my personal health journey?

...................................................................................
...................................................................................
...................................................................................
...................................................................................
...................................................................................

5. What's holding me back from getting better faster? List as many words, emotions, and thoughts as you want.

....................................................................................
....................................................................................
....................................................................................
....................................................................................
....................................................................................
....................................................................................

6. What is it going to take for you to jump the line? Get out of sick care to true personal "health" care?

....................................................................................
....................................................................................
....................................................................................
....................................................................................
....................................................................................
....................................................................................

7. What's the opportunity cost of not getting better? What would you lose by not even considering or making a change from your current path? What's the cost of staying sick?

................................................................................
................................................................................
................................................................................
................................................................................
................................................................................
................................................................................

8. What would life look and feel like if the transformation already happened? Picture how you look, what you'd wear, how you'd move, how you'd feel, what your environment looks like, what your food looks, feels, and tastes like, who's around you, what activities, how does work look and feel different?

................................................................................
................................................................................
................................................................................
................................................................................
................................................................................
................................................................................

# LESSON 8:
# MINDSET TO MIND GROWTH

*"Believe you can, and you're halfway there."*
-Theodore Roosevelt

Consider this: patients who received placebo treatments, believing they were real medicine, experienced genuine relief in up to 40% of cases across various conditions[3]. This remarkable insight highlights the effectiveness and significant role our mind plays in our health journey.

Our thoughts and beliefs, often operating in the background, play a larger role in our recovery than many realize. In this chapter, we'll delve into the role of mindset and how it can help (or hinder) your recovery.

Imagine this: your mind is the conductor, and it's orchestrating your body's health. Every cell, like members in an orchestra, is listening, watching, waiting for direction, following its lead. As the conductor triggers certain sections to begin playing, other sections ready themselves because they know the patterns; their part comes next. It's not just a whimsical notion; it's grounded in solid scientific research. Our thoughts, our stories in our head, and our words with our internal dialogue send

[3] https://www.nejm.org/doi/full/10.1056/NEJM200105243442106#:~:text=Placebos%20have%20been%20reported%20to,as%20pain%2C%20asthma%2C%20high%20blood

intangible and tangible mental currents flowing through our daily lives and hold the key to our physical well-being. Like an orchestra will always follow its conductor, the body always follows the mind.

Dr. Gabor Maté, a physician, speaker, and author well known for his work in the fields of addiction, mental health, and the mind-body connection, has written extensively on topics related to the impact of early childhood experiences, trauma and stress on physical and mental health in the adult. He has focused his lifelong work on understanding the link between emotional and psychological factors and various symptoms and diagnoses.

He suggests conditions such as autoimmune diseases and chronic pain may be linked to emotional stress and trauma. He argues that chronic stress resulting from adverse childhood experiences may lead to an overactive or dysregulated immune response, potentially increasing the risk of autoimmune diseases like multiple sclerosis. He believes that unhealed childhood trauma can contribute to various mental health issues, including anxiety, depression, and addiction. It's not just his observation but mine as well that when you observe a waiting room full of ALS patients, there is a smile, happiness, even forced happiness, and a desire to make others happy on their faces.

My mother had ALS, and I still remember her forced smile most of the time. Is there a link in the thought pattern of someone who's the ultimate people pleaser or cheerleader that alters the immune system to start and fuel someone's path to certain disease states like ALS or multiple sclerosis and other disease states? The answer for me is a resounding yes.

For many years with my own autoimmune diseases and treating thousands of people with autoimmune diseases as well, I noticed a common thought pattern: we all struggled with a lack of forgiveness. I have an incredibly hard time forgiving myself and others. This has led me to ask questions of those with autoimmune diseases if they indeed struggle with knowing how to forgive and that it is a major pain point in their emotional lives; the answer very often is yes.

How powerful is the mind? Why does one person endure a high level of pain while another has such a high pain perception that even a small injury produces a high level of pain? Thoughts influence our perception of pain levels. Have you noticed that when you're feeling low, aches and pains seem to come out of nowhere or are worse? Or, in a desire to not rock the boat or make anyone else bothered, you endure more pain and put on a smile? You know, if you had to, you can focus on something else or try to ignore the pain, and that can change how much pain you feel.

I have noticed that when I'm feeling very emotionally overwhelmed, I lose my voice and struggle to get my voice out. Do you notice that when you encounter certain situations, a particular part of your body has pain associated with someone, somewhere, or a situation? The mind, the memories, the stories, and the thoughts influence the function and symptoms of all our body thoughts.

The power of positive intention. The placebo effect is when someone experiences real measurable improvements in their symptoms or condition after receiving a treatment that has no actual therapeutic intervention. For example, there is no active medication, but a person believes that they took something that had medical activity. It's a measurable response that occurs simply because someone believes they took something they thought would be beneficial.

The placebo effect can range from 30-60% improvement of a symptom, depending on which study you read. This is more effective than most medications on the market today. The placebo effect has been well studied to help in medical conditions, including pain management, depression, anxiety, and even Parkinson's disease. So all it takes is your mind to have thoughts that this will work, and it does 30-60% of the time across studies. That's a very powerful result.

All this points to how the body will follow the mind. So if we are to have changes in our bodies and we are looking for changes in our symptoms or diagnosis, the most important thing first is to look inwards, towards our mind.

## Step 1: Raise Your Level of Awareness

What are my thoughts? What are my stories? Many people don't think about the connection between their thoughts and their symptoms. So, I want to offer some tools right here to help you connect your thoughts or stories with a particular symptom or medical problem you have.

What are the words I'm using towards myself, my body parts, my beliefs? For example, this damn shoulder keeps bothering me. She stabbed me in the back when she stole that money. I can't stomach another word from him. I have a broken heart. Why do I have to shoulder everything? This person is a pain in the neck. I'm such a mean person. I'm a klutz. I'm a broken person.

Were the words yours? Were you told that you were a pain in the neck? That you were a waste of time. Were you told that you are clumsy or mean? Were you born with those words speaking inside of you? Who told you that? Who put that thought or words into you?

In our lives, we often carry the weight of words and perceptions from the past. Reflect on a particular belief about yourself and trace it back to the very moment it was implanted.

For instance, my first memory of being labeled a "troublemaker" was at age seven, during an unforeseen incident.

Left in charge of three other kids, an unexpected fire broke out. My instinct was to ensure their safety and alert the neighbors to put out the flames. Yet, the aftermath was a storm of blame directed at me. My father's silence lasted two weeks. This label haunted my steps, leading me through both my youth and adulthood with a self-image tainted by guilt. Consequently, I felt responsible for everything and everyone, consistently overburdening myself, which culminated in grueling 60-hour work weeks throughout my twenties. Perhaps it's no surprise that I wrestle with persistent shoulder pain.

If you were told you were a bad seed, would you feel qualified to be a mother? How do the repeated words and thoughts, I'm a bad seed affect one's ability to conceive or mother a child? How would that trigger lifelong feelings of aloneness, being blamed, and being overly responsible for others? How would that impact your perception of your own pain and your pain tolerance? How would that impact someone becoming a workaholic to have some worth and value to others?

All of this from an experience as a child with a fire where the words and thoughts were implanted by someone else, "It's all your fault. It's always all your fault. You will have to be always responsible for every problem, failure, or death that will occur because you're a bad seed." This is an example of a powerful story, a very traumatic experience with huge emotional pain points that forever establish neuropathways. And as you read the words above, could you feel your own emotional response and physical response start to happen? The effects and stories of trauma leave indelible patterns that persist through life and turn into diseases.

These words were not ours. These thoughts were put into us. My parents, in my example, were doing the best they could with good intent. But that experience did create and start my lifelong problems with pain and my high tolerance for it. It did create a thought pattern of ignoring or diminishing my own pain while feeling overly responsible for the experiences of others.

In the programs I've developed, it's critical that people understand this concept of the body following the mind. Without work to change the patterns of the mind first, no physical transformation can happen in their health. This is why one of the first exercises we work on is raising our level of awareness around our stories. Often, we don't even realize these stories are programs running us.

So, I've provided a list of thought-provoking questions for you to consider and work on to raise your level of awareness around your thoughts, stories, words, and where they really came from.

For example, the belief, the generalization that "nobody likes me." This can expand into beliefs like, "If anyone actually really knew the real me, they'd never truly like me."

Does that sound like you? Or find another belief you have about yourself, and really, let's examine and question it with the following questions.

- What are the words I'm using to describe myself, my body, my beliefs?
- Are these words mine? Who or where did they come from?
- What is my earliest memory of the person who said these words first to me?
- What is the story I associate with this word or thought?
- What are the emotions that I associate with this story?
- What are the beliefs that came out of this story about me?

## Step 2: The Pattern Interrupt

A pattern interrupt is a psychological technique that serves as a deliberate and strategic disruption of recurring thought patterns, emotions, or behaviors. These patterns of thought often become automatic and ingrained, sometimes leading to unproductive or negative outcomes. For example, the recurring belief that you're a klutz may actually produce a self-fulfilling prophecy where, in fear of injury and obstacles, you run or move in a way as to protect yourself from injury but are actually in a hunched posture with a tight fist and forearms with your body tilted forward.

This pattern of protection on your body may lean you forward chronically, causing you to be more prone to tripping, falling, and spraining your ankle or knees. It can also lead to your shoulders rolling forward to protect your chest, leading to a chronic state of recurring shoulder and chest pain. This is a belief you have that's caused a physical pattern of holding your body and in movement that creates more injury and chronic pain.

The purpose of a pattern interrupt is to break free from these entrenched patterns, creating a pause or shift in thinking that allows for increased awareness and the opportunity for change.

One example of a pattern interrupt is the physical action method. Imagine you are about to go on a run, and you're already thinking, "oh no, I'm a klutz; what if I trip and fall again?" While running, you find yourself repeatedly scanning the ground ahead, adjusting your steps to avoid obstacles. This preoccupation keeps you from truly enjoying the run. Realize this repetitive cycle every time you head out; try suddenly clapping your hands. This abrupt noise and physical action can serve as a jolt to your current thought pattern.

It forces you to momentarily shift your focus from the anxiety-inducing thoughts to the sensory experience of clapping, disrupting the loop of anxious thinking. This physical clap of your hands can also include a few seconds of you doing a fist pump or a dance. You may start your music with a song that makes you feel invincible.

The physical sensation of the sound, the clap on your hands, the fist pump, or the dance snaps you out of a common pattern. You take sound further and play a song that makes you feel strong, confident, and energetic, and the pattern interrupt has worked.

Another example is mental imagery. If you find yourself ruminating on a past mistake, you can use mental imagery to interrupt the pattern. Imagine before you a bright red stop sign flashing in your mind's eye whenever these thoughts resurface. This mental image functions as a huge neurological reset button from the vision to the rest of your brain and body to interrupt unproductive thoughts and redirect your attention. It's like erecting a mental barrier that prevents you from going down the same mental path, giving you space to think differently and more constructively.

Within our programs, I often liken both myself and participants to puzzle solvers. When I notice someone trapped in a particular mindset—expressing sentiments like, "My achievements aren't as big as Jane's, but..." or "I know I have a long way to go, but..." or even "I should've known better; this is my fault"—it's evident that their narrative revolves around feelings of inadequacy, comparison, and self-blame. While I care deeply and often may be too emotionally involved, my primary aim is to help them recognize these patterns.

The transformative power of experiential learning is on full display when others hear such statements. As observers, we can often see reflections of our own past behavior in others, fueling empathy and understanding. I recall Jane once shared a similar sentiment, which now serves as a reminder for me to be mindful of my own tendencies towards negative self-comparison.

When we identify these patterns in participants, we inquire if they're receptive to us highlighting these tendencies. By mirroring their words back to them, a moment of realization often ensues. Hearing your own self-deprecating words from someone else's mouth is a powerful wake-up call. Many participants, upon hearing their words echoed back, have remarked, "I am too harsh on myself. I need to shift my mindset." After all, if you wouldn't direct such criticism towards others, why subject yourself to it?

Awareness is the first step. While some might initially lack this self-awareness, our programs aim to elevate it, spotlighting these self-limiting beliefs and behaviors. While it can be uncomfortable to hear our own words reflected back, it's a vital tool to challenge and change deep-seated thought patterns. After all, can true health and life transformation occur without first altering our perceptions and the language we use? This mental and emotional evolution forms a cornerstone of our experiential journey.

To help you create your own pattern interrupts, here is a guideline:

1. Surprising and unexpected: the element of surprise is essential to be effective. These thought patterns are coming on autopilot, and your brain and body are already on a roll. To break this cycle, you need something unexpected. It could be as simple as making a sudden noise, like clapping your hands or breaking into song or dance. Or it can be funny and unexpected images that take your brain off guard. I have a GIF I won't share with you but every time I see that thing, I burst out laughing uncontrollably. Find a funny image in your head or thoughts.

2. Engages the senses: incorporate sensory experiences like touch, sight, or sound. Carry a small item in your pocket, like a gem or coin, that has a unique texture, color, and weight. Touch it when you want to interrupt a thought pattern. This tactile sensation can ground you and shift your focus in a second.

3. Quick and easy: the best pattern interrupts are those you can do quickly and effortlessly. They don't require a lot of time or planning either. Keep it simple. Simple actions or mental images that can be executed in seconds work the best. A pet rock in the pocket, a snap of the fingers, a rubber band on your wrist to snap, or a click of your tongue. There's no need to overthink it.

4. Align with your values: the best patterns are ones that align with your personal values and goals. They should shift your thinking toward those goals in a positive and constructive way. For example, if your goal is to reduce stress, the pattern should be one that promotes relaxation and mindfulness, like a smooth gemstone with your favorite color in your pocket to touch and meditate with. If your goal is more playfulness in your life, you should have a power pose that reeks of fun to you when you feel uptight or stuck. I've got one, what's yours?

Pattern Interrupt Creation:
1. The pattern that I want to interrupt. Think when this thought or situation happens, it's a downward spiral.
2. What are some ideas of things I can do that will engage my senses, like touch, sight, or sound, that I can do in that situation?
3. Is it quick and easy? If not, how can I make it quick and easy?
4. Does it align with the result I'm trying to achieve? If not, do I need to think of another option?

## Step 3: From Mindset to Mind Growth

One of the most powerful things to do once you're aware of the thought patterns and you've learned how to interrupt them is to start thinking about how you can change those words, stories, and beliefs permanently. This is thought transformation. Do you want to change the thought or story permanently?

What's the mindset? Mindset is the mental framework shaped by your past experiences, childhood beliefs, and personal traumas. We've discussed in the section about raising your level of awareness that the questions there are designed to bring to the surface the subconscious mind to the conscious. What are the words, the stories, the who's, and the beliefs that shaped the thought patterns that trigger physical illness?

Being aware is the first step, and the ability for quick pattern interrupts helps quickly pause or shift the focus. But the ultimate result you really need is the power to change those thoughts and stories permanently. Mind growth is a transformative process that involves challenging and changing old stories, beliefs, and words. This process leads to the development of new thought patterns and behaviors and an overall expansion of one's potential. You can't have a new physical transformation without the shift to the mind growth transformation.

There is the uncomfortable beauty of transformation. Imagine the journey of a grub inside the chrysalis, metamorphosing into a butterfly, is nothing short of a miraculous odyssey. At first, it finds itself in a chrysalis of discomfort, surrounded by a mushy, formless existence. This stage, often unglamorous dubbed the "mush phase," is where the real magic happens. The grub's body undergoes a profound change, shedding old skin and structures that once defined it.

As the transformation unfolds, it encounters moments of turbulence and instability. It's as if the universe itself is challenging the grub's very essence, pushing it to its limits. The once-familiar contours are gone, and in their place, an entirely new form begins to emerge. Yet, it's not a graceful transition; it's a gritty, transformative battle where old identities and limitations are shattered.

In the midst of this chrysalis chaos, the grub experiences a profound metamorphosis, pushing past its own discomfort and the boundaries of its former self. And then, one day, it emerges, its wings unfurling like fragile poetry, revealing a resplendent butterfly, reborn in beauty and grace. It's a testament to the incredible power of transformation—a reminder that growth often emerges from the most uncomfortable and challenging of cocooned spaces.

Transformation happens in this uncomfortable, mushy, gritty, scary environment. This grub has to push past its own physical and mental limitations. It was to want to grow and change. It's pushing its boundaries against its cocoon. It's painful as new legs and wings push out around its body. There is a battle to stay as it is. This is the environment you want to get into and embrace. You have to want the transformation so badly that you're willing to be in this uncertain, dark, yucky, challenging space. This is the only place true transformation can occur.

This is precisely the transformation that happens in the mind growth work that people experience when they play full out for themselves in our programs working with me. I do challenge their old words, thoughts, stories, and beliefs. I invite them to start learning how to live in that space to start doing that with themselves. I truly understand that no other doctor or medical program has invited them to do this uncomfortable level of growing and challenging their minds. I would not ask anyone to do work I'm not willing to do and have done myself. I also wouldn't ask someone to do something that wasn't effective and necessary.

I continue to operate in this uncomfortable, challenging space of growth for myself and my clients. What I know for sure is this. I am certain without any doubt that had I not embraced mind growth over the past decade; I would never have had the transformation to be a happy, healthy, thriving person with a new lease on my life.

Everything that's happened to me has happened for me. It's in this space of discomfort that I keep expanding my own limits and keep getting better, not only for my own physical and mental health but in my role as a teacher and doctor.

## 8 Steps of Mind Growth

1. Recognize the comfort zone
2. Embrace the challenges
3. Seeking discomfort
4. Embrace failure as a learning opportunity
5. Cultivating a growth-oriented mind
6. The beauty of transformation
7. Overcoming the fear of change
8. Celebrating growth milestones

This is definitely a topic for another 8 Out-of-the-Box book. But I wanted to give you a glimpse of the courageous and vulnerable work that happens with clients who work with us. It is a fact that the reason why we have such successful health transformations is that the people who are attracted to working with us understand they want and crave mind growth. They know it's the tool that's been missing all along, and it holds the key to their physical transformation, innately if not overtly at times.

Our initial lesson revolved around "Leading with Curiosity." It encouraged you to venture outward, seeking fresh questions and their intriguing answers.

Now, this lesson circles back to the same theme, but with a twist: we're channeling that curiosity inward. We're diving deep into your mindset, unearthing old narratives, thoughts, and beliefs that may have cemented patterns of ill health over time.

In this concluding lesson, my aim is to arm you with the tools necessary to heighten your self-awareness. We'll transition those deep-seated patterns from lurking in the shadows of your subconscious to the spotlight of your conscious mind. Moreover, I introduced you to the game-changing technique of a "pattern interrupt."

To wrap up, my final gesture is to guide you on a transformative journey—from a stagnant mindset to a thriving mind growth. Here, in this fertile ground of mental expansion, we'll bid farewell to outdated beliefs, welcoming the enriching discomfort that nudges us towards fresh horizons—new acquaintances, skills, behaviors, and convictions. This is where you truly break free and embrace profound transformation.

## Action Steps

I've provided a list of thought-provoking questions for you to consider and work on to raise your level of awareness around your thoughts, stories, words, and where they really came from.

- What are the words I'm using to describe myself, my body, and my beliefs?

..................................................................................
..................................................................................
..................................................................................
..................................................................................
..................................................................................
..................................................................................
..................................................................................
..................................................................................
..................................................................................
..................................................................................
..................................................................................
..................................................................................
..................................................................................

- Are these words mine? Who or where did they come from?

..................................................................................
..................................................................................
..................................................................................
..................................................................................
..................................................................................
..................................................................................
..................................................................................
..................................................................................
..................................................................................
..................................................................................

- What is my earliest memory of the person who said these words first to me?

..................................................................................
..................................................................................
..................................................................................
..................................................................................
..................................................................................
..................................................................................
..................................................................................
..................................................................................
..................................................................................
..................................................................................
..................................................................................

- What is the story I associate with this word or thought?

..................................................................................
..................................................................................
..................................................................................
..................................................................................
..................................................................................
..................................................................................
..................................................................................
..................................................................................
..................................................................................
..................................................................................
..................................................................................
..................................................................................
..................................................................................

- What are the emotions that I associate with this story?

..................................................................................
..................................................................................
..................................................................................
..................................................................................
..................................................................................
..................................................................................
..................................................................................
..................................................................................
..................................................................................
..................................................................................
..................................................................................
..................................................................................

- What are the beliefs that came out of this story about me?

..................................................................................
..................................................................................
..................................................................................
..................................................................................
..................................................................................
..................................................................................
..................................................................................
..................................................................................
..................................................................................
..................................................................................
..................................................................................
..................................................................................
..................................................................................

## Pattern Interrupt Creation:

- The pattern that I want to interrupt. Think when this thought or situation happens, it's a downward spiral.

..................................................................................
..................................................................................
..................................................................................
..................................................................................
..................................................................................
..................................................................................
..................................................................................
..................................................................................
..................................................................................
..................................................................................
..................................................................................

- What are some ideas of things I can do that will engage my senses, like touch, sight, or sound, that I can do in that situation?

..................................................................................
..................................................................................
..................................................................................
..................................................................................
..................................................................................
..................................................................................
..................................................................................
..................................................................................
..................................................................................
..................................................................................
..................................................................................
..................................................................................

- Is it quick and easy? If not, how can I make it quick and easy?

..................................................................................
..................................................................................
..................................................................................
..................................................................................
..................................................................................
..................................................................................
..................................................................................
..................................................................................
..................................................................................
..................................................................................
..................................................................................
..................................................................................

- Does it align with the result I'm trying to achieve? If not, do I need to think of another option?

..................................................................................
..................................................................................
..................................................................................
..................................................................................
..................................................................................
..................................................................................
..................................................................................
..................................................................................
..................................................................................
..................................................................................
..................................................................................
..................................................................................
..................................................................................
..................................................................................

# CONCLUSION

Congratulations, you've gone through a journey of the eight biggest lessons to experience in order to jump-start your health transformation. To start any journey, you need to start by **Leading with Curiosity.** Do you ask the right questions of yourself and others?

The five W's of curiosity-based questions:

- Who?
- What?
- Where?
- Why?
- When?

Most importantly, it is not a question but a statement of: tell me more.

When you lead with these questions, even a simple but difficult-to-solve problem like pain or constipation can lead to answers, directions, and people that you'd never imagined before. These questions lead to experiences that change your health from sick to true personal health care.

In **Digestion - The First Domino**, we begin to understand how a sequential order of approach is essential. It's the critical first system that food and nutrition come into that's ignored.

You learned about all the parts of this system and how they work together. We also introduced the role of supplementation. Learning why and how supplements work and when they are and are not needed is critical.

**Gut microbiome and Infection** is a huge problem, and this highlights the lesson about why order matters. No other lesson is more on point than this one. I would recommend not focusing on infection first when it's the victim of other processes going wrong before it. Definitely think about digestion, blood sugar, food sensitivities, detoxification by the liver and fermentation problems before pursuing infection. We do have programs in Transform that help people end infection. However, we do this by helping them gain the know-how and the experience of cleaning up their gut environment first. This must be what happens to ensure an effective infection eradication if needed in the future. No more merry-go-round with your gut.

Why stop there? **Certainty About Food** does matter, but testing is adequately maligned and poor. Food Mapping is available in our Transform Program; however, one of the dreams of our company is to keep growing and developing new experiences. One of the areas we'll be growing into is rolling out more live experiences, data, education, and transformations in the area of food and nutrition. Get on our email list and join our Facebook group. I want you to be the first to know when we have a new experience coming to you, in person or virtually.

In the lesson about **Blood Sugar Mastery**, you learned how many common symptoms are the tell-tale signs of blood sugar fluctuations. Using insomnia, brain fog, pain, histamine issues, and POTS as major symptoms that are data points, your body is talking to you about the state of blood sugar in you. It's critical to understand the data your body is providing you. And you can use tools like bookending the day to save the day.

The lesson on **Hormones** truly highlights the lack of training and the misaligned financial considerations that go into why hormonal imbalances are at epidemic levels. And there's something you can do about it. We'd love to have you get the data, virtual education, and live training and create the experiences you need to manage your hormones for life in MY Hormone MasterClass.

If experiences are what you know you need for Transformation. I invite you to understand the kinds of experiences needed for health transformation. I discussed in the lesson **Creating Experiences** the types of experiences that are critical but absent from the healthcare landscape. I discussed the role of data, virtual education, live medical training, movement, community, and mindset to mindgrowth work. If any of that resonates with you, reach out and talk to us!

The pinnacle of our experiences is about transforming your **Mindset to Mind Growth**. My hope is that this book has empowered you to open your mind and your thoughts to new approaches, new ideas, and new outcomes. I hope I've challenged you in some of your mindset thinking about your health and your life. I hope it opens Pandora's box in excitement and focus.

One of my core values is fun. Whatever experience we have in life, in order for it to have an impact, it's got to be fun. I'm inviting you to join the fun and excitement that happens every day in Transform. We are live on social media; there are books and workshops happening regularly. There are podcasts and new YouTube videos we're sharing about people's experiences. The people on the team at Transform and the clients in Transform are busy living our best lives. We create impact in our own lives, and we hope to inspire others to do the same.

Book a call with our team at Transform. We want to learn more about you and where in your life and health you feel like you need some help. We have many different types of experiences, from books, to workshops, to virtual programs and live events to fit anyone.

We work with individuals who are ready to be active drivers of their health transformation. People who are curious, excited, and fun to work with. People who want to experience and live life to their fullest.

People who will invest themselves in experiences as that is the only way for transformation. People who are ready to change the trajectory of their lives for themselves and their families. Is that you? Let's connect!

Fast-track this by scheduling a chat with one of our team members

www.drmaggieyu.com/apply-bk

# ABOUT MAGGIE YU MD IFMCP

Dr. Maggie Yu, a dedicated functional medicine physician, has become a force to be reckoned with in the world of functional medicine. An author, mother, teacher, speaker, and thought leader. Her journey has been anything but ordinary. Battling her own debilitating health challenges, she recognized the limitations of conventional medicine. This profound personal experience became the catalyst for a career-altering deep dive into alternative methods of healing.

A visionary in her field, Dr. Yu's transformative approach combines the best of medical knowledge with holistic care. The result? The Transform System. A groundbreaking protocol that has not only transformed her life but has also proven to be a beacon of hope for countless others suffering from similar afflictions. It goes beyond treating symptoms; targeting the root causes of health challenges to bring about lasting change.

In this book, you will discover more than just Dr. Yu's medical expertise. You'll gain insight into her resilience, dedication, and unwavering commitment to redefining health care. Dr. Yu believes in empowering her patients and equipping them with the knowledge and tools they need to take control of their health. With an array of resources, tools, and supportive strategies, she presents her protocol not as a mere alternative but as an essential game-changer.

For anyone on the cusp of losing hope or simply seeking a better understanding of their health, Dr. Maggie Yu is the guide, mentor, and ally you've been waiting for. Dive into her story, embrace her wisdom, and embark on a journey to vibrant health and wellness.

**Coming soon to the series:**

- 8 Out of the Box Companion Guide to Transformative Recipes
- 8 Out of the Box Ways to Transform Mast Cell Activation & Histamine Intolerance
- 8 Out of the Box Ways to Transform Your Hormones

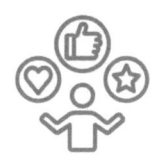

# EXPERIENCES AVAILABLE THROUGH TRANSFORM

I want to invite you into a system of experiential learning to transform your health.

## Transform Fundamentals Program

Want to turn around any chronic illness whether you have a diagnosis or not? This program is ideal for individuals with autoimmune diseases of every kind. Ideal for difficult-to-treat diagnoses like fibromyalgia, POTS, Dysautonomia, Mast Cell Activation and Histamine Intolerance, and long haul with COVID-19. People who struggle with complex symptoms without a specific diagnosis, like chronic fatigue, chronic infections, neuropathy, and chronic pain, have successfully worked with us to experience total health transformations.

- A virtual experiential learning program that utilizes a client's own unique data to comprehensively master the root cause triggers of disease.
- They work directly with our medical team, which includes a physician, functional nutritionists, hormone experts, mind growth experts, movement experts, and alumni mentors to get direct live expert guidance on implementation.
- Content and curriculum include a focus on personal growth and gaining powerful tools to interrupt physical patterns to transform them into new patterns

of wellness. I teach the Five Pillars of Transform as a root cause approach to healthcare and thoroughly explore for each person. You can check out the Five Pillars of Transform in the training below.

- There is engagement within a community while working in small groups with alumni mentors to create accountability and support. The program creates therapeutic relationships within the program and with providers outside the program that last a lifetime.
- Clients learn more by watching the training below and booking a call with our team so we can learn more about your needs. Pairing the right person with the right program is critical to their success.
- Additional programs available to alumni of Transform Fundamentals.

To learn more about the Five Pillars of Transform to discover your root causes, watch this training
https://go.drmaggieyu.com/start-now

To turn around any chronic illness or symptom, book a call with our team
www.DrMaggieYu.com/Apply

To deep dive into the program and case studies, subscribe to our YouTube channel
https://www.youtube.com/@DrMaggieYu

# MY Hormone Masterclass (MYHMC)

Staying awake all night, hot flashes, anxiety, pain, brain fog, weight gain? Hormonal hell can hit anyone at any time.

The problem is it's hard to know the right time or the proper test. It's even harder to find a provider that will test your hormones. And even if you got the hormones, do they understand the results to show you the hidden patterns that are making and keeping you sick?

Enter Dr. Maggie's MY Hormone Masterclass. This is our wildly popular hormone program, where you get to be in charge.

- Get the right test sent directly to your home
- Know the exact time to get accurate results
- Learn the hidden patterns of hormone imbalance even your doctors or naturopaths don't even know about
- Get live expert guidance from medical hormone experts directly in live review sessions
- Clients can work with us for one review session or up to a year with unlimited sessions to continue to balance their hormones.

To learn more, check out:
www.MyHormoneMasterclass.com

## MY Food Mapping

Over the past years, the biggest request was for us to offer the Food Mapping System to every person who wants clarity in their food reactions. I'm pleased to announce that we are introducing it during the first quarter of 2024.

- If you or someone you know suffers from seemingly random reactions to food? Have you been to the allergist and have been told it isn't related to food allergy? Yet you know that it is food that you're reacting to, but it's impossible to understand why you're reacting to some foods sometimes while at other times you may not. In the chapter **Certainty About Food is Required**, we dove into why I created the Food Mapping System to bypass all the bad tests, bad advice, and bad outcomes people have.

- Get the right test directly sent to you and your family

- Learn through online video modules all the different ways besides allergies that you could be reacting to food.

- A full year's access to the learning modules to be done at your own time and your own pace.

- Understand digestion and its impact on your food reactions.

- Understand what are false positives and negatives on your test results so you know it's 100% accurate.

- A one week review session with our team to review results and get the nutritional support you need.
- The ability to add-on family members so everyone can get clarity and results.

To learn more, check out
www.MyFoodMapping.com

## MY.MD Bio-Therapeutics

Dr. Maggie created a supplement company designed to address the root triggers of any chronic disease. With a mission of outcome-driven supplementation, an emphasis is placed on a minimal number of high-quality ingredients that have been scientifically studied to produce results.

The supplements and medical food referenced in this book can be found at: www.mymdshop.com

To learn more about supplementation, watch the library of training videos available on
www.youtube.com/@mymdshop

## Additional Experiences

Virtual workshops and events
Upcoming live events near you

Stay up to date by making sure our emails are in your inbox, and add our email address to your trusted list of contacts. Join our Facebook group. Subscribe to our YouTube channels.

# APPENDIX

## Balancing Meals

### Breakfast

- 2 eggs, scrambled/fried | serve with 1-2 cups of sauteed vegetables like broccolini, mushrooms, sweet/spicy peppers, kale/hard/spinach + sausage, bacon, smoked trout/salmon, avocado for added protein and fat
- GF Steelcut/Rolled Oatmeal | 1 serving is 1/2 cup dry oats, 1/2 cup mixed seeds and nuts, 1/4 cup berries, 1/4 cup kefir/yogurt
- High protein vanilla chia pudding

### Lunch

- Pro-collagen WB Smoothie | 1 scoop Pro-collagen WB, handful of green avocado, almond or coconut milk or cream, 1/2 cup fruit, Pro-MCT C8 oil, manuka honey, monk fruit, or Stevia to sweeten
- Super Green Protein Salad | top with sardines/lunch meat/meat leftovers (great with feta cheese, avocado and lemon vinaigrette
- Quinoa and Bean Bowl with cilantro lime dressing and avocado

## Dinner
- Lentil Soup with Sausage and Chard (in recipe book)
- Roasted chicken thighs (skin on and bone in) with fennel and red potatoes
- Slow cooker Thai beef stew over quinoa
- Bratwurst/Italian sausage with grated sweet potatoesand greens
- Sauteed shrimp (4oz) and collards/chard with sun-dried tomatoes

## Snacks
- 1/4 cup pumpkin seeds and 1/2 apple, jerky, celery and nut butter, hummus and carrots
- Avocado with lime, cilantro and hard-boiled egg

# Blood Sugar Balancing: Daily Meal Planner

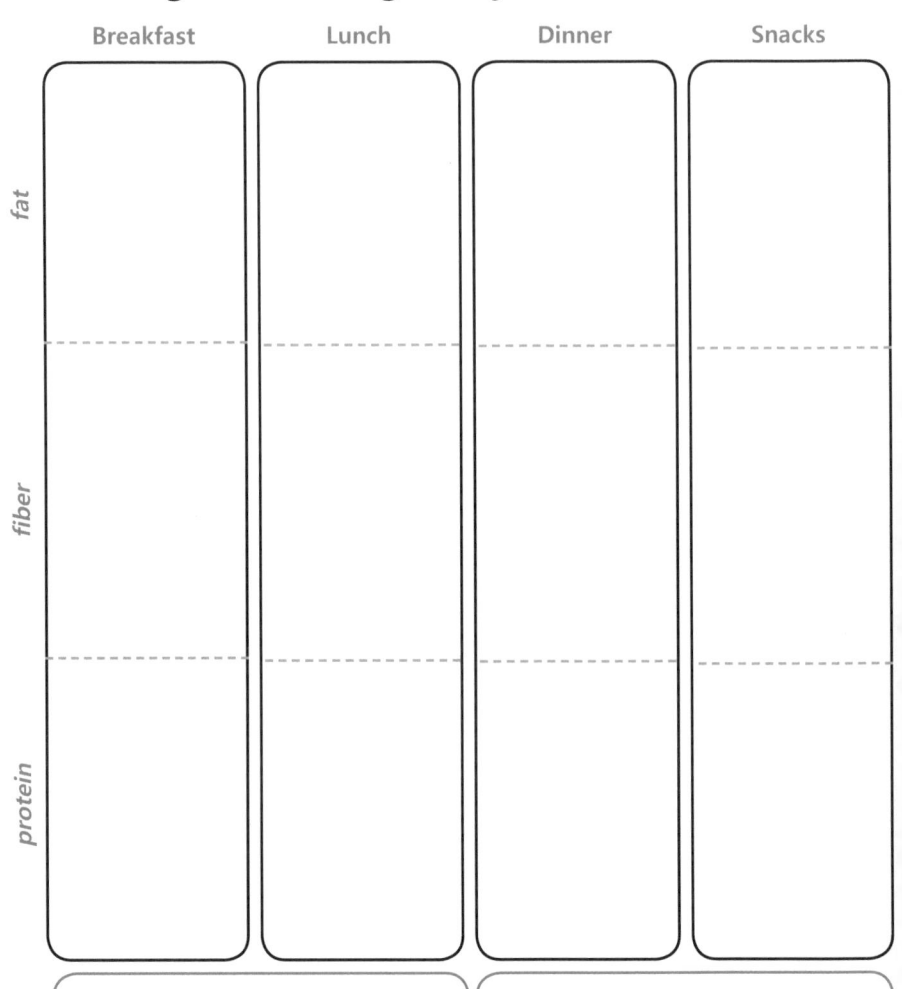

|  | Breakfast | Lunch | Dinner | Snacks |
|---|---|---|---|---|
| fat |  |  |  |  |
| fiber |  |  |  |  |
| protein |  |  |  |  |

**Batch cooking ideas:**

**Blood Sugar Regulation - stay ahead of the hunger!**

- eat within 1 hour of waking
- all meals/snacks are balanced
- bookend the day with protein
- eat every 3-4 hours

**8 Out of the Box Ways to Transform Your Health**
From Confusion to Confidence: The Playbook for Whole Body Wellness

# Gluten Free Meal Plan

|  | Monday | Tuesday | Wednesday | Thursday | Friday | Saturday | Sunday |
|---|---|---|---|---|---|---|---|
| **Breakfast** | Breakfast porridge with berries | Potato with chard and leek scramble | Potato, feta, tomato and basil fritata | Potato, feta, tomato and basil fritata | Rice kimchi, greens and an egg | High fat green smoothie | Gluten-free pancakes with bacon and berries |
| **Snack** | Endurance crackers with anchovies | Almond butter and apple | High fat green smoothie | Endurance crackers with anchovies | Hemp seed protein bar | Hemp seed protein bar | Chia seed pudding |
| **Lunch** | Rice and beans with mango salsa | Quinoa salad | Kale with maple glazed tempeh and miso dressing | Southwest chicken soup | Vegetable hummus wrap | Quinoa salad | Leftover tray bake on top of mixed salad greens |
| **Snack** | Vegetable with hummus | Chia seed pudding | Almond butter and apple | Chia seed pudding | High fat green smoothie | Vegetable with hummus | Hemp seed protein bar |
| **Dinner** | Rosemary roasted chicken with potatoes and simple salad | Chicken tacos with quick slaw | Southwest chicken soup | Fish and roasted tomatoes | Prok chop, blackeyed peas and greens | Tray bake with salmon | Beef/elk/lamb burger with guacamole and roasted potatoes |

# Grocery List

**Produce:**
- Berries
- Mango
- Apples
- Bananas
- Lemons
- Limes
- Garlic
- Avocados
- Mixed Salad Greens
- Basil
- Parsley
- Rosemary
- Cilantro
- Onions
- Carrots
- Celery
- Jalapeno
- Cherry Tomatoes
- Roma or Beef Steak Tomatoes
- Fingerling or Red Potatoes
- Fresh or Frozen Spinach
- Ginger Root
- Leeks
- Beets (pickled, or make your own)

**Pantry:**
- Unsweetened Coconut Flakes
- Dates or other dried fruits
- Pumpkin Seeds
- Flax Seeds
- Chia Seeds
- Walnuts
- Sunflower Seeds
- Sesame Seeds
- Poppy Seeds
- Hazelnuts or Almonds
- Hemp Protein Powder
- Garbanzo Beans
- Black Beans
- Anchovies
- Full-Fat Canned Coconut Milk
- Psyllium Seed Husks
- Dijon Mustard
- Apple Cider Vinegar
- GF Otameal
- Tahini
- EVOO/Coconut Oil
- Almond Butter
- Rice
- Kimchi
- Quinoa
- GF Tamari
- Rice Vinegar
- Blackeyed Peas
- Gluten Free Wrap
- GF Corn Tortillas

**Meat and Cold Items:**
- Eggs
- Feta Cheese
- Tempeh
- Miso Paste
- Non-dairy Milk (Cashew, Flax, Almond, etc,)
- Whole Chicken
- Salmon
- Ground Beef/Elk/Lamb
- Pork Chops
- White Fish

**Seasonings:**
- Salt
- Pepper
- Cinnamon
- Cumin
- Corriander
- Paprika
- Garlic Powder
- Onion Powder
- Vanilla Extract
- Maple Syrup, Stevia, etc.

> **MEAL PREP**
> We recommend planning one day a week to shop, prep and batch cook!
>
> For this meal plan, you should prep ahead.
>
> Wash and chop all vegetables.
>
> Hummus, Endurance Crackers, Hemp Seed Protein Bars, Chia Puddings

8 Out of the Box Ways to Transform Your Health
From Confusion to Confidence: The Playbook for Whole Body Wellness

# RECIPES

## High Fat Green Smoothie

Zip, boom, bang! This smoothie brings a flavor jam and blood sugar balancing act to life.

### INGREDIENTS:
- 3/4 cup coconut milk or coconut cream
- 1¼ cups water
- 2 - 4 Tbsp lime juice
- 2¾ oz. frozen spinach
- 1 Tbsp fresh ginger, grated

### PREPARATION:
- Blend all ingredients together. Start with 2 tablespoons of lime juice and increase the amount to taste.

### TIPS:
Prep your smoothies ahead of time to ease the morning rush. They last in the fridge for up to 2 days. Use an airtight lid, and remember to shake well before drinking!

# Protein Smoothie

Use this as your go-to morning or snack smoothie. Change it up by subbing the banana for 1/2 cup servings of another fruit.

## INGREDIENTS:
- ½ can coconut milk
- 1 banana (or sub 1/2 cup other fruit)
- Handful of frozen berries
- 1 to 2 tbsp protein powder or nut butter
- 1 raw egg (optional)
- Handful of spinach

## PREPARATION:
- Put the banana in a blender (optional), add coconut milk, followed by all other ingredients. Blend until smooth and enjoy.

## TIPS:
Freeze your over-ripe bananas for extra creamy and cold smoothies. Peel ripe bananas. Then, break it in half or cut it into small discs. We recommend freezing it on a parchment paper lined sheet pan before placing it in a ziploc bag.

# Rice, Kimchi, Greens And An Egg

**INGREDIENTS:**
- ½ cup kimchi
- 1 cup leftover, long grain rice
- ½ bunch chard
- 1 leek, sliced thinly
- 2 garlic cloves, minced
- ½ lemon, juiced
- 1 egg
- 1 Tbsp EVOO
- Sea salt to taste and fresh ground pepper

**PREPARATION:**
- Chop chard stems about ¼ inch thick.
- Combine chard stems, leeks, pinch of sea salt, fresh ground pepper and EVOO in a medium stainless steel pan. Saute at medium heat for about five minutes.
- Add chard leaves and garlic to the pan. Saute for 5 more minute, squeezing in lemon toward the end.
- Heat leftover rice.
- Pan fry egg over easy.
- Combine in bowl with eggs, greens, and Kimchi on top

# Kimchi

Fermentation time: 7-14 days | Makes: 1 Quart

## INGREDIENTS:
- 1 large head Napa cabbage, cut into bite-sized pieces
- 2 baby bok choy, cut into bite-sized pieces
- 3 large carrots, grated
- 1 daikon radish, julienned
- 1/2 of an onion, thinly sliced
- 1 apple, grated
- 5 scallions, cut into 1-inch pieces
- 7 cloves garlic, peeled
- 3 inch; piece of ginger, peeled and cut into pieces
- 1/4 to 1/3 cup crushed red chili flakes, depending on how much heat you like
- 1/4 cup fish sauce (optional if you want to make it vegan)
- 1/4 cup unrefined sea salt

## PREPARATION:
- In a very large bowl, add the Napa cabbage, bok choy, carrots, daikon radish, apple, scallions, and onion.
- Add the garlic, ginger, and red chili to a food processor. Process until it forms a paste. Add this paste to your big bowl of vegetables.
- Add salt and fish sauce to the bowl and massage everything with your (clean!) hands for 4-5 minutes until the vegetables start to break down and there is liquid forming at the bottom of the bowl.

- Transfer the kimchi to one very large clean jar (or a couple of clean smaller jars), making sure to pack the vegetables firmly, submerging them in brine. Make sure to leave at least 1 inch of free space at the top of the jars before securing the lids.
- Leave the jars out on your countertop or in your pantry for a few days, periodically unscrewing the lids slightly to let out carbon dioxide. Also, I made sure to push the vegetables down under the brine with a clean fork every other day.
- After 3 days, you may begin to taste your kimchi. I liked the way mine tasted after 7 days, but feel free to let it go longer to get it really sour. When it is good and tangy to your liking, transfer the jars to the refrigerator, where the kimchi can keep for months.

# Coconut Fat Bombs

## INGREDIENTS:
- 1 package of unsweetened shredded coconut
- 1/2 cup coconut oil, melted (can add a little less/more for texture)
- 1 1/2 to 2 tsp flavor extract of your choosing (vanilla, almond, lemon, maple, etc)
- Filling mixture (lemon zest, baked apples with cinnamon, dried fruit, nuts, etc.)
- Almonds (or nut of choice)

## PREPARATION:
- Take a package of unsweetened shredded coconut and dump it into a food processor with the blade in place. This is how you make homemade coconut butter. You can also buy it already made in stores, but this is a less expensive and simple way to make your own.
- Blend until the coconut is soft and fluid, 4-5 minutes.
- With the processor running, add some melted coconut oil, enough to make the mixture liquid enough to pour.
- Add a flavoring extract.
- Scraping down the sides of the food processor with a spatula, transfer the mixture to a measuring cup to make it easier to pour.

- Pour into mold (You can use whatever molds you want, i.e., mini muffin pan lined with liners, silicon shape molds, etc.)
- Fill each mold with a filling of your choice, + 3 almonds in each.
- Gently pour the coconut butter mixture into each cup, being careful not to overfill them.
- Put the tray in the fridge or freezer for a few minutes to set.

# Cabbage Slaw

The perfect balance of crunch and tang to detox your liver while adding a zesty side dish to any meal.

## INGREDIENTS:
- 1 bunch green kale washed, ribs removed and finely sliced
- 1/2 napa or other savoy cabbage, finely sliced
- 1/2 cup shredded carrots
- 1 cup cilantro, chopped
- 1/4 cup ACV or lime juice
- 2 Tbsp olive oil
- Salt and pepper to taste

## PREPARATION:
- Place kale, cabbage and carrots in a large bowl
- Add cilantro last
- Dress with ACV and EVOO
- Add salt and pepper to taste
- Let sit to wilt cabbage slightly

# Chia Seed Pudding

Makes 3 servings.

## INGREDIENTS:
- 1/2 cup full-fat coconut milk
- 1/2 cup non-dairy milk (almond, cashew, flax, etc.)
- 1/4 cup chia seeds
- 1 Tbsp maple syrup, honey, or agave (optional)

## PREPARATION:
- Mix all wet ingredients together, then add chia seeds. Stir.
- Wait a few minutes until the mixture begins to thicken. Add more liquid if desired.
- Divide into 3 small jars, cover and refrigerate.
- Let sit at least 20 minutes before serving. It will keep in the fridge for 3-5 days.
- Put the tray in the fridge or freezer for a few minutes to set.

## TIPS:
Before serving, top with fresh berries, cocoa nibs, or shaved coconut.

# GLOSSARY

**Ankylosing spondylitis:** A type of inflammatory arthritis affecting the spine and sacroiliac joints. It causes back pain and stiffness.

**ADD (Attention Deficit Disorder):** A neurodevelopmental disorder characterized by difficulties with attention and concentration. It's often diagnosed in childhood and can persist into adulthood, affecting daily activities and cognitive functions.

**ADHD (Attention Deficit Hyperactivity Disorder):** A neurodevelopmental disorder marked by persistent patterns of inattention, hyperactivity, and impulsivity. While similar to ADD, ADHD includes the hyperactivity component. It's commonly diagnosed in children but can also be recognized in adults.

**ALS (Amyotrophic Lateral Sclerosis):** A progressive neurodegenerative disease that affects nerve cells in the brain and spinal cord. Often referred to as "Lou Gehrig's Disease," it leads to the loss of muscle control, affecting movement, speech, and eventually, breathing.

**Autonomic dysfunction:** Problems with the autonomic nervous system, which controls involuntary functions like heart rate and digestion. It can cause dizziness, fainting, and more.

**BALANCHER:** A supplement containing berberine, cinnamon, and chromium to help regulate blood sugar and insulin levels.

**C. difficile:** Also called Clostridioides difficile, it is a bacteria that can cause symptoms like diarrhea and abdominal pain, often after antibiotic use.

**Crohn's disease:** A type of inflammatory bowel disease causing inflammation and damage in the digestive tract.

**DAO (Diamine Oxidase):** An enzyme that breaks down histamine.

**Dysautonomia:** A blanket term for various disorders affecting the autonomic nervous system. It can cause dizziness, fainting, fast heart rate.

**DIGEST-IT:** A multifaceted digestive enzyme supplement created by Dr. Maggie Yu. It contains ingredients to support all steps of digestion.

**Epstein-Barr virus:** The virus that causes mononucleosis ("mono"). It can also cause chronic fatigue.

**Estrogen dominance:** A hormonal imbalance where estrogen levels are abnormally high relative to progesterone levels.

**Fibromyalgia:** A condition characterized by chronic widespread pain and tenderness. Fatigue, sleep issues, and depression are common.

**Food Mapping System:** A system developed by Dr. Maggie Yu to accurately test for and identify food sensitivities and intolerances. It involves education, testing, and guidance.

**Gastroparesis:** A condition in which the stomach has delayed emptying, causing nausea, vomiting, and other symptoms.

**GOLDEN BALANCE:** A medical drink containing collagen, turmeric, and herbs to help balance blood sugar overnight. Created by Dr. Maggie Yu.

**Graves' disease:** An autoimmune disease and common cause of hyperthyroidism, leading to overactivity of the thyroid gland.

**H.pylori:** Also called Helicobacter pylori, this is a bacteria that infects the stomach and can cause ulcers, gastritis, and stomach cancer.

**Hashimoto's disease:** An autoimmune disease that affects the thyroid gland. It is the most common cause of hypothyroidism.

**HbA1c:** A blood test that measures average blood glucose levels over the past 2-3 months. Used to diagnose diabetes.

**HISTAWAY:** An enzyme supplement containing DAO to degrade ingested histamines from food allergies.

**HRT (Hormone Replacement Therapy):** Administration of hormones like estrogen or testosterone to counteract hormonal decline.

**Hypothyroidism:** A condition in which the thyroid gland is underactive and doesn't produce enough thyroid hormone. Symptoms include fatigue, weight gain, dry skin, and depression.

**IBS (Irritable bowel syndrome):** A common gastrointestinal disorder causing abdominal pain, bloating, and changes in bowel habits.

**Leaky gut syndrome:** Increased intestinal permeability, allowing substances to leak from the gut into the bloodstream, potentially triggering inflammation or autoimmunity.

**Lipopolysaccharides (LPS):** Toxic bacterial compounds released when bacteria die, contributing to inflammation.

**LIVER LOVE:** A liver support supplement containing milk thistle, alpha lipoic acid, NAC, and other ingredients to optimize liver function.

**LOVE MY GREENS:** A nutritious greens powder supplement delivering phytonutrients from vegetables and antioxidant fruits.

**LOVHER:** A supplement containing liver and hormone-balancing ingredients like calcium d-glucarate, DIM, and green tea extract.

**MCAS (Mast Cell Activation Syndrome):** An immune disorder causing allergy-like symptoms triggered by certain foods, medications, and chemicals.

**Menopause:** The natural end of a woman's menstrual cycle, marking the end of fertility. Perimenopause refers to the transitional time leading up to menopause.

**PCOS:** Polycystic ovary syndrome, a hormonal disorder causing irregular periods, infertility, and other symptoms.

**Neuropathy:** Nerve damage causing numbness, tingling, weakness, and pain in the extremities.

**Ox bile:** Bile salts derived from oxen that can supplement bile production to aid fat digestion.

**Polymyalgia rheumatica:** An inflammatory condition causing muscle aches and stiffness, especially in the shoulders.

**POTS (Postural Orthostatic Tachycardia Syndrome):** A condition in which heart rate increases abnormally upon standing, causing dizziness and other symptoms.

**Prebiotics:** Non-digestible fibers that promote the growth of beneficial gut bacteria.

**Probiotics:** Live beneficial bacteria and yeasts that confer health benefits when consumed.

**PRO-COLLAGEN WB:** A powdered collagen supplement from Dr. Maggie Yu to support healthy skin, hair, nails, joints, and gut lining integrity.

**PRO-FLORA AI+:** A targeted probiotic supplement to support immune health and intestinal microbiome balance.

**PRO-FLORA GI:** A probiotic supplement containing the studied LP299V strain to improve gut health and digestive function.

**PRO-OMEGA 1000:** A high-potency fish oil supplement providing omega-3 fatty acids EPA and DHA. Helpful for heart, brain, and hormone health.

**Raynaud's Phenomenon:** A condition that causes reduced blood flow to the fingers and toes, typically triggered by cold temperatures or stress.

**SCFAs (Short chain fatty acids):** Produced by gut bacterial fermentation, which provide energy and other benefits.

**SIBO (Small Intestinal Bacterial Overgrowth):** Excessive bacteria in the small intestine causing symptoms like bloating and diarrhea.

**Sjögren's Syndrome:** An autoimmune disease affecting moisture-producing glands. It causes dry eyes, dry mouth, and other symptoms.

**Trigeminal neuralgia:** A chronic pain condition affecting the trigeminal nerve in the face, causing intense facial pain.

# PERSONAL ACTION PLAN

**Page Number**     **Notes**

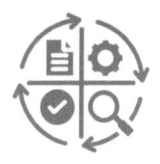

# PERSONAL ACTION PLAN

**Page Number**  **Notes**

# PERSONAL ACTION PLAN

| Page Number | Notes |
|---|---|
| | |